# Sleeping with COVID

ఞ ఞ ఞ

## A True Story of
## Despair Inside a COVID Ward

By

*RJ Charest*

<u>This book is dedicated to:</u>

"Thank you" to the Care Givers and First Responders all over the world who are placing their life on the line every day helping others manage their terrifying struggle with COVID-19.

Copyright © 2021 RJ Charest.

All rights reserved. No part of this publication may be reproduced, distributed, or transmitted in any form or by any means, including photocopying, recording, or other electronic or mechanical methods, without the prior written permission of the publisher, except in the case of brief quotations embodied in critical reviews and certain other noncommercial uses permitted by copyright law.

- ISBN 9798504594545

- Cover design by Author

- Book layout by Author

- Printed by Amazon KDP

- Page count 91

- First printing edition 2021

**Disclosure:** Actual names were changed to protect the privacy of individuals. Any similarity is coincidental.

This book was written for entertainment use only and should not be considered as medical guidance. Please seek a licensed medical professional for medical advice.

# Contents

# Introduction

The planet is under siege by a new breed of biological creature never previously documented! Earths landscape still looks the same but the society that lives within lives in fear of the killing power of these new creatures. Previously, cancer was the feared killer of humans. Now the new king of killers' sports multiple crowns atop its body and is so tiny it cannot be seen by the naked eye and yet over the past year it has killed more humans than anything on earth.

The science researchers identified these tiny creatures and placed them in a virus category with the name "SARS-CoV-2" but the US population uses a slang version COVID or COVID-19 with 19 meaning the virus discovery year 2019.

Did these creatures travel the universe to get here or did they naturally evolve on earth? More sinister tales are that mankind made them for biological warfare and they escaped? Discovering the origin of COVID-19 is no small task, but a worthy effort for a future Nobel Prize.

This is a true story of grandpa getting run over by COVID-19 on New Year's Day and the travesty that follows in an overcapacity healthcare system. Experience the terror of three severe COVID cases documented bedside in a hospital COVID ward. Warning, check your dignity at the emergency entrance!

# Chapter One:  Happy New Year

It is New Year's Eve 2020 and the world over families celebrate with traditional meals believed to usher in luck for the coming new year. Not unlike this pair… Patty and Ron a New Jersey couple who met through online dating and now happily living together. Both recently retired and spent most of 2020 at home hiding from the deadly world pandemic lurking outside.

It is 4 pm New Year's Eve 2020 and Patty announces she is going to start preparing the holiday meal. Ron skipped lunch today, except for a few holiday cookies, to save room for the feast. Patty spent two hours the day before just ordering groceries online and fighting the busy home delivery system for available delivery times. Patty found some fresh jumbo shrimp to use in a shrimp alfredo, but the homemade sauce is her secret handed down from her mother.

The kitchen slowly fills with the smell of roasted garlic, Ron's mouth waters… and asks Patty if she needs any help. Patty urges Ron to take charge of selecting and serving the wine for the feast. Ron finds a three-year-old bottle of Barbera they made together at a wine school and uncorks the bottle. The wines nose is pleasant, so a taste is poured… its good but edgy and needs to breathe a bit so into the decanter it goes.

Patty notices Ron back in front of the TV and pipes… "You can help with the salad if you're not busy." "On it" Ron replies. Patty preps the garlic butter for the garlic knots, another of Ron's favorite special occasion indulgences. Ron chops the salad using a new set of

Pampered Chef salad choppers that his mom and sister just sent as a Christmas gift. Earlier in the day, Patty cleaned her inherited china and now sets the dining table which is fit for royalty.

## The Traditional Feast

The formality of the feast begins with Ron helping Patty get seated. Wine glasses are raised and a farewell bid to 2020 is called "clink." Patty voices her hopes that 2021 will get back to normal, no lofty expectations… only normal would be nice! Ron agrees and grabs the breadbasket and finds a garlic knot to chomp into. Mmmmm! With warm knowing glances, silence prevails as the New Year's Eve feast is consumed.

The wine is bold in taste, the creamy shrimp alfredo is delicious, and the broccoli perfect al dente. Ron compliments the chef, "another feast well done dear." He takes a small second helping and a fourth garlic knot and surmises, "I could happily make a meal of the knots and a glass of wine." The meal being so filling… a dessert was not prepared, but Christmas cookies are still abundant in this house. Patty lovingly calls Ron "Cookie Monster."

Relaxing in a gluttonous daze… both look forward to the normalcy that 2021 promises with the COVID vaccine finally beginning distribution. Patty wants to see more of her grandbabies and Ron hopes to travel to Florida to spend time with his mother and sister. Both look to spend more public time together at the shore. Patty sits back in her chair, a 'full' tell that Ron recognizes. Ron grabs his wine glass and toasts Patty, professing his love for her in which she returns the favor… clinking!

## Farewell 2020

With the feast cleanup complete Patty and Ron settle in front of the TV. It is 7 pm in New Jersey, London is celebrating midnight and the arrival of their New Year. The UK is also on pandemic lockdown so, no public gatherings, but the BBC is broadcasting previous firework shows and songs from safely sequestered entertainers. The majestic Big Ben clock face in London is shown chiming loudly, hence ringing in the new year. Ron flips around the channels and they watch some American entertainers. By 10 o'clock Patty yawns and announces she needs to head to bed, but Ron is feeling uncomfortably full and chooses to stay up.

Well past midnight Ron pulls himself up from a slumber on the couch. His stomach yields mild pain, but he passes it off as overindulgence and recent couch potato posture. Cookie Monster entertains the thought of having bedtime cookies, then the notion is pushed aside once reason kicked in. Ron turns off the Christmas lights around the house, reflecting… this may be the last lighting for the season. "Happy New Year!" he mumbles.

Ron opts for a quick shower in hopes of washing off the final 2020 funk. Lathering up he notices his belly is distended and grabs ahold, "Too many Christmas cookies Cookie Monster!" and laughs. New Year's clean, Ron heads to bed.

## A New Year 2021

It is New Year's morning and a sharp stabbing abdominal pain startles Ron awake. Seems his tummy ache has turned ugly as he slept. He feels around the stomach and no amount of rubbing or prodding relieves the pain. Thrashing about does not seem to help either. Its 4:12 am and Ron decides to get up and sit in a recliner so as not to wake Patty. Some more pressing and pushing reveals that the source of the pain is located under the right-side ribcage.

Ron is that guy the physicians hate… a Google self-diagnostic. So, the research begins. It does not take long to identify the organs in that area and decides it is most likely the gallbladder. Four plus years ago during an unrelated chest scan the medical technicians identified some stones in his gallbladder. The physician consensus then was "If the stones are not a bother, then do nothing until they are bothersome." Well bothersome they are now. Ron begins his several hour investigative journey into reading everything gallbladder and gallstone related.

Dawn is breaking, 6:12 am New Year's morning, and Patty appears quietly from the shadows of the hallway. Softly she asks Ron, "Are you okay?" Ron replies, "I think not!" Ron explains his pain level as a nine causing shivers and nausea. Patty suggests they seek help, and Ron concurs and adds a "New Year babe!" wish, less the Happy part. Both proceed to get dressed for the journey.

## Pandemic Angst Builds

Ron contemplates his decision to seek help in a hospital harboring many sick COVID patients. He shakes at the thought or was it the sharpness of the pain? He read online that if one waits too long and the gallbladder bursts the results can turn catastrophic quickly. So, wait-and-see does not seem to be an option here. But Ron does wait for Patty to get ready. His heart races over the angst of visiting a hospital during a pandemic with no other options.

Over the past ten months the daily news channels pushed COVID fear to the public. Broadcasts display charts with staggering numbers of infected and disturbing death rates around the world. Warnings to stay away from public spaces. Ron's stress level is off the charts over this decision to visit a hospital. He and Patty have been so good with sheltering in place up to this point in time. Ron pleads "God, please wake me from this nightmare!" Patty's reappearance jolts Ron from the darkness of his mind… it appears this is real… the transport is dressed and ready to make the journey.

Patty starts her weeks old car and asks Ron, "How do you feel now?" Ron replies, "queasy!" Patty returns to the house and reappears with a bucket and a towel and places them in Ron's lap. Patty asks, "Do you need anything else?" Ron replies, "a hospital!" Off they go.

It is 6:45 am now and the drive to the hospital is 19 minutes according to the GPS. Ron apologizes to Patty for getting her up so early. Since retirement both enjoy sleeping in. The new car smell is making Ron nauseous and he fights back the urge to be sick! Ron is back to internally stressing over the hospital visit. Patty asks, "Are you sure you want to do this?" Ron replies, "No… but I see no other choice, it being New Year's morning!"

The hospital appears on the horizon and it towers above the surrounding landscape like an alien ship crashed in the suburbs. A shiver shakes Ron again stemming from a fear of hospitals, a pain, a chill or both he is not sure. The emergency entrance is clearly marked, and Patty parks at the drop off. They kiss, and then Ron pulls up his facemask and departs saying, "I will call you." Patty cannot come inside due to new COVID security rules, so she heads back home.

## Hospital Intake

Walking towards the emergency entrance Ron focuses on numerous signs posted on the door. "Not a Visitor Entrance" and "Masks Required at All Times Inside the Building". Ron adjusts his mask and presses on. The entrance and reception area are quiet with no other patients at 7:08 am New Years day. The firework patients with lost fingers are already inside being tended to. Upon entrance, Ron is greeted by the entrance guard Jack who would rather be anywhere but here. Jack promptly blocks Ron's path and asks if Ron is here for COVID treatment. Ron replies, "No, not COVID related" and is then directed to the registration desk where Nancy collects driver's license information, insurance information and reason for visit.

Ron is then directed to an intake room off the reception area where patient vitals are also recorded. Ron is thankful for the quiet environment of the entrance where only hospital workers can be seen and not the crowds of people in waiting rooms he had envisioned.

Damien, a jovial young man and intake lab technician, seats Ron then himself at a computer screen and asks Ron for his name and date of birth. Damien indicates Ron has answered correctly and proceeds to print a barcoded wrist band and affixes it to Ron's wrist while joking "all the girls will be jealous." Damien takes Ron's vitals… blood pressure, heart rate, temperature, oxygen levels and records them. Ron is also asked some mental health questions. Damien blurts out, "Now I got it, you look like Kurt Russell… do you get that a lot?" Ron: "No, but that can't be bad, right?" Damien: "You must get all the girls." Ron: "Just the best one!"

Hospital policy mandates that all patients submit to a COVID test during intake. Damien pulls a long Q-tip from a sealed package and instructs Ron to remain still while he swabs Ron's nose. Ron is brought to tears by the deep penetration of the procedure and chuckles, "That tickled my brain!" Intake complete, a wheelchair and driver Terrell appear, and Ron is instructed to climb aboard.


## Closer Inspection

The trip is short to a nearby small room with a diagnostic table and Terrell instructs Ron to climb onto the table. Terrel indicates, "Someone will be in shortly to perform a preliminary diagnosis, please remain on the table." And exits the room.

Twelve minutes pass and Doctor Whitacre enters the room and identifies himself to Ron as an M.D. Ron is again questioned on what brings him in today. Ron describes his abdominal pain and indicates the primary location. Dr. Whitacre feels about Ron's abdomen asking if differing pressure hurts. Ron explains his four-year prior diagnoses of having Gallstones. Dr. Whitacre pushes about more and says, "I am going to have an ultrasound done on your gallbladder, please remain here."

A short time later, lab technician Brittney enters the room pushing a cart with a portable ultrasound. She announces, "I will be taking some images of your gallbladder today." Brittney apologizes for the coolness of the lubricant she is applying to his abdomen. Ron's pain level is already a 9 so Brittney's pressing of the imaging probe on his belly does not increase the pain level. Imaging complete she indicates, "The doctor will have a look at the results and be back shortly to discuss."

It is a long wait... Ron looks at his phone, no cell service. He knows Patty will be expecting updates and writes a text explaining he is still in intake, then presses send knowing the phone will send the message once service is reestablished. 8:24 am, Dr. Whitacre returns to the room carrying the test results and describes the diagnosis, "You have a serious infection in the gallbladder so you will be admitted to the hospital. Transport will be here shortly to take you to a room."

## Royal Transport

Jamal arrives with a wheelchair to transport Ron to his assigned hospital room. The awaiting wheelchair is the king of wheelchairs built to carry 400-pound patients with ease. Jamal is a friendly and talkative young man. He loads Ron while constantly chattering and grinning. Along the way Jamal is welcomed back by many of his coworkers as he passes them in the hallways. Today is Jamal's first day back to work after fighting a battle with COVID and all the red tape required to come back to work after recovery. Today he loves his job!

Ron and Jamal round a blind corner, no mirrors, and bump feet to feet into another transport on a hospital bed. The patient, a middle-aged woman in the cancer ward is expressionless over the encounter. Ron says, "woo… want to play footsies?" Still nothing… Ron wishes he said nothing.

Arriving at Ron's room Jamal comments, "wow, your lucky day… you got a single room, not many of those around here." Nurse tech Karen enters the room and directs Ron to get onto the awaiting hospital bed. Jamal spins his chariot and exits the room with a hushed song and a swagger in his stride. Karen gets Ron settled on the hospital bed and gives instructions about bed operation and the emergency call devices attached.

## Getting Settled In

Ron stares at the ceiling and tries to relax. A large clock on the wall indicates that it is 9:15 am. Ron assesses his pain level as an 8 but wonders if he is just getting used to the level 9 pain. He checks his phone again, one bar now and the earlier text was sent. One bar will not permit a phone call, so he sends Patty another text update.

Ron's room is right in front of the nurse's station and he imagines that could be helpful. He also notices there is no in-room bathroom and decides that is a big negative. More shivers over the thought of using a bed pan. Pain sure causes a lot of shivers! The bed controls provide Ron with some amusement and needed distraction.

A cart rolls into Ron's room seemingly by itself. Looking closer it's a noticeably short Hermosa pushing the cart. She announces she is here to take Ron's vitals.

Hermosa takes Ron's arm and wraps the blood pressure cuff, then clips on another heart rate and oxygen monitor. She pulls a wired thermometer from a holster and starts for Ron's mouth. Ron jumps with a "wow, where has that thing been?" Hermosa explains the holster disinfects the thermometer, but she can also put on a thin plastic cover if Ron wishes. Ron shivers and replies, "No thanks!" Hermosa replies, "I can also take your temperature from your armpit." Ron responds, "If you don't have a heat gun then okay." The collected vitals appear on the cart screen and Hermosa indicates, "all looks good."

## Giving Blood

Luciana, a blood lab technician arrives in Ron's room and announces that she is here to take blood. Ron groans… and warns Luciana that he is a hard stick. A medical community slang term for a person that is difficult to draw blood from. Ron has small rolling veins, and for added difficulty, his veins are deeper under the skin than most. Luciana has a year of doing this fulltime, so she has heard plenty of whining before.

This hospital has a two-stick maximum per technician or nurse. Meaning that a person only gets two tries to extract blood. After two tries they must stop and leave the patient. The next try on the same patient must be performed by a different technician and at least an hour later. Luciana is on her second try and beginning to fish around, meaning she missed the vein on this last try and is twisting the needle to try and snag it. Ron knows his rolling veins will escape her fishing attempt and asks Luciana to stop as it is painful. Luciana packs up her supplies without a word leaving Ron baffled as he is not yet aware of the two-stick rule.

Ron has a building urge to urinate, and at 72, he knows the perils of waiting too long to seek relief. Still green on the hospital protocols Ron gets out of bed and sticks his head out the door. A nurse at the station says, "You must remain in bed, can I help you?" Ron replies, "bathroom?" The nurse points to a corner in the hall and says, "Use that one." Ron with his street clothes on feels comfortable, no butt hanging out, while strolling down the hallway to the bathroom.

It's now 10:50 am New Year's morning and another blood technician Fanibhusan arrives announcing the need to take blood. Ron explains to the technician that he is a hard stick and wondered why the last tech left without drawing blood. This is when the two-stick rule is explained to Ron. Fanibhusan takes Ron's arm and begins to slowly stroke towards the hand while looking closely at the inner arm. The technician concurs, "deep!" He manages to hit the vein on the first try and easily extracts two vials of blood. Ron commends Fanibhusan on a job well done. Fanibhusan returns the compliment with a departing bow.

## More Testing

A lab technician, Logan appears in Ron's doorway and announces he is there to collect COVID-19 test samples. Ron indicates, "That was done three hours ago during intake." Logan replies, "I do not make the decisions as to who gets what, I just collect the samples based on an order request." Nurse tech Karen reentered the room and assures Ron that the doctor orders all tests. Ron protests again saying, "How could the original results change over the past 3 hours unless I was infected during the trip to the room." Karen explains the three-to-five day COVID-19 incubation period, where a recent infection can take three to five days before a test will recognize the infection. So, a recent infection will not show up on the new test. Now a retest makes even less sense to Ron. He is exasperated but submits to the second test while mumbling "This is why my healthcare insurance costs so much!"

Ron makes another trip to the bathroom and finishes with some cold water to the face in hopes of relieving some stress. He returns to his room and moans while climbing onto the hospital bed. Any twisting of his trunk results in a sharp stabbing pain in the abdomen. Ron's at rest pain level is still a painful 8. He also notices the pain is now radiating up his lower back and thinks to himself, "That cannot be good… calm down Ron."

Candice, a sleep lab technician studying to be a nurse enters the room with Ron's CPAP machine which he ordered during intake. The machine is four times the size of his home machine and sits atop of a sturdy rolling table. Candice asks, "Which side of the bed?" and Ron prefers his left side. Candice hands Ron several size masks to choose from and he selects the medium size. He opens the sealed mask and tries it on and gives it a thumbs up. Candice asks Ron for his pressure setting, and Ron being a twenty-year home user knowingly responds with, "Eleven." Candice enters the pressure setting and shows Ron the power button he will use to turn the machine on and off. Candice asks, "any questions?" Ron replies, "Nope, thanks."

## Test Results

It has been twenty-five minutes since the COVID test and Karen returns to the room. Karen informs Ron that the test results are back with a COVID-19 positive result. They must move him again and the transport is en route. A look of terror consumes Ron's face! He stammers, "what?" And Karen repeats the bad news. Ron demands a recount, "It is my right to have a tiebreaker test… it is 1 to 1 now!" Karen indicates that Ron will have the opportunity to discuss that with the doctor. Ron asks, "Where am I moving to?" Karen responds, "The COVID ward." Ron realizes he is now hyperventilating and tries in vain to recompose. Ron demands, "Then… then I need to speak with the doctor before the move!" Karen responds, "The doctor is not on the floor at this time." A feeling of complete despair numbs Ron, and a darkness surrounds him, feeling faint Ron blurts out, "I'm going to die here!" Karen replies, "You can refuse treatment and we release you." Ron, "I can not do that either, it is too risky to let the gallbladder go untreated." Karen, "Transport will be here soon."

The news media and health experts over the past ten months relentlessly pushed the fear of how deadly COVID is to the elderly. Ron at age 72 fits the elderly high risk of death category. He and Patty both knew they were high risk, so they diligently followed all CDC precautionary guidelines.

Ron reflects on the countless stories in the news of senior center outbreaks and the high death toll within those groups. Ron's focus shifts to Patty, thinking if he has COVID then Patty must as well! Ron fumbles to text Patty but transport arrives before he can do so.

## Off to See COVID

It is Jamal who returns at 1:07pm as Ron's transport. Jamal greets Ron, "My man, it's you… where are we going this time?" Ron responds, "Hell!" Jamal replies, "Dang, this bus don't go dare!" Cheerful Jamal helps Ron into the chair and off they go. Ron works on his text to Patty filled with uncharacteristic obscenities and incomprehensible gibberish. Tears running down his face as he writes and ignores Jamal's attempts of cheerful chatter. Ron gasps, he cannot send this to Patty and deletes the message.

The COVID ward is on the first floor so another long ride. Ron contemplates his options… he really wants to leap from the wheelchair and run for the hospital exit. But he has a painful gallbladder ready to rupture so just leaving will not solve anything. If he remains in the hospital, a COVID infection is inevitable providing he is not already infected. The results of a single test returning a false positive changed Ron's future and possibly his longevity. Ron has none of the symptoms of a COVID patient and feels wronged by the hospital now holding him captive in a no-win situation.

It will be hard for Ron to grasp this concept… once a person tests positive for COVID in the healthcare system they are treated as such for the near future regardless of any offsetting tests. Only a successful fourteen-day quarantine, free of COVID symptoms changes that designation. Ron's gallbladder will not wait fourteen days.

## Welcome to The Hive

Exiting the elevator on the first floor and a short distance down the hallway Ron and Jamal stop at a large, closed double door. The borders around the door are marked with brilliant yellow hashes with black background. The doors are adorned with multiple red lettered signs indicating, "Warning Infectious Disease Ward", "Authorized Personal Only" and "No Visitors". Jamal swipes his badge, and the double doors swing open. Ron exclaims, "Gates of Hell… it's real now!" Jamal concurs, "Dang bro, you were right!" Jamal stops his cheerful chatter realizing the source of Ron's mood change from earlier. Jamal is a COVID survivor and can relate to the pain and suffering in this ward. Ron's long forgotten gallbladder pain is replaced by the terror of what he is about to do… Sleep with COVID!

Moving beyond the "Gates of Hell" the hallways look the same as the other side. Ron's mind reels with dark thoughts… "I've entered a COVID hive!" He recalls the first sight of the hospital building resembling a crashed alien ship. He Surmises, "This is the belly of that ship." Behind each door they pass are human hosts, each breeding COVID hives within their chest. These hives release fresh COVID virus into the air from the lungs of their captured humans. The humans are such easy prey and perfect hosts with their warm moist lungs. The hallway seems dimmer now. Ron fidgets with his mask as he fights the despairing thought of himself becoming a host!

## The Welcoming Committee

Jamal stops at door 106 and announces, "Here we are… we will wait here for a nurse." A few seconds pass before nurse Bonnie appears followed closely by her tech assistant Cassa. They are the welcoming team ready to place Ron in his room. This is a two-bed room as are all the COVID rooms.

Ron now realizing he will have a roommate implores with Bonnie; "Can I get a single room? I am willing to pay the difference!" Bonnie replies, "There are no single rooms in this ward honey... only doubles." Ron releases a long exhale in despair and mumbles a faint expletive.

Hospital staff must suit up each time before entering a COVID room and remove and dispose the gear upon exiting. They first apply a second mask over the mask they already wear and pull-on protective gloves. They then pull on a yellowish green jumpsuit over their scrubs then place a hooded shield over their head. They look like a NASA team ready for a spacewalk.

Ron is placed in the far bed and is walked past Andre in the first bed and introductions are made. Ron says "Hello" and Andre grunts back. Ron's hospital bed is the same type as the previous room, so he lowers the bed himself to easily climb in. Cassa hands Ron the call for service remote and the TV remote. Each patient has a TV, Cassa asks if Ron wants the TV on and he replies, "No thanks." The curtain between Andre and Ron is pulled some to give each privacy.

Ron looks at his phone, Patty sent several text messages asking how he is doing. Lost for words Ron returns a muted response. How does one explain this debacle in a text message? Other family members and friends also sent text messages. Texting helps pass the time and each second spent texting is one less spent thinking about the hopelessness of the situation.

## Stick it Rule

Nurse Bonnie indicates she needs to insert a port on Ron's arm so they can begin an antibiotic drip for the gallbladder infection. Ron groans and informs Bonnie of his misfortunate status of being a hard stick. Bonnie's first attempt fails and after Ron watched the first attempt closely, asks Bonnie to look deeper for the initial stick. Bonnie's second attempt is successful, and she secures the port to Ron's arm, then attaches him to the IV pump. She agrees with Ron being a hard stick as she rarely misses the first try. Ron comments, "I like the two-stick rule here" just to confirm its existence in this ward. Bonnie, an older wiser nurse indicates they would not need that rule if the people doing the sticking were trained better. Rule confirmed!

Vitals are taken twice each shift and they are most annoying when the midnight shift takes theirs at 1:00 and 5:00 in the morning. Triana "Anna" collected Andre's vitals while Bonnie worked on Ron's port. Now it is Ron's turn for vitals. Anna is a young mother of two and is uncomfortable being in the Infectious Disease Ward, but technicians must rotate servicing all locations within the hospital. Anna likes her job but servicing this ward triggers a mild anxiety attack, so she breathes deep to work past the building stress. Anna knows the COVID spores travel in the air so breathing deep triggers more anxiety after just working on Andre who does not wear a mask.

The vitals technicians obtain their service instructions from a wireless tablet carried by each technician. The tablet transmits each patients' vitals to a central computer making the data immediately available to the doctors and other hospital staff members. Vitals outside of the normal range generate alerts to hospital staff.

Anna preparing to take Ron's temperature pulls the wired thermometer from her cart and aims for Ron's mouth. Ron startles Anna with a "Whoa! You just pulled that thermometer out of my roommates' highly infectious mouth and now you want to stick it in my mouth? That is never going to happen! In what reality is that a good idea?" Anna assures Ron the machine sanitizes it between uses, but also indicates she can take his temperature from his armpit. Ron still protests, "I really don't want that near me" Anna, "I cannot force you but monitoring your body temperature provides a first warning that you may be fighting COVID-19. I can put a plastic shield on the thermometer and take it from your armpit." Ron reluctantly agrees, "Go ahead, put a condom on it and I will have safe COVID!" Anna covers the thermometer with a disposable plastic shield and takes Ron's temperature. Ron is flabbergasted that they would reuse oral test instruments or any instruments in an infectious disease ward. That is like saying, "Here… take a taste of COVID!" Perhaps they assume everyone here has COVID, Ron still does not have COVID-19 symptoms. He believes it was a false positive test result that put him in this ward.

Ron's vitals are normal except for his now-elevated blood pressure and his heart rate is above normal which is a change from earlier readings. Anna explains the vital numbers to Ron while struggling to project her voice from behind the bulky headgear she is wearing. She nervously adjusts her headgear and departs in a hurry.

Anna, like most hospital workers, comes home each day to a family. They must protect their families from the horrifying environment in which they work. Anna, just prior to arriving home calls her spouse to sequester the children before she enters the apartment. Anna then enters and goes directly to a bathroom and takes a long shower and puts on clean clothes. Dirty laundry is placed into a disposable plastic bag and immediately placed into a washer. Anti-bacterial lotion is everywhere in the house. Temperature checks also occur often in Anna's household.

## Andre the Giant

Andre, Ron's roommate, is a 46-year-old Jamaican from Hanes. He has a large body type comparable to a chubby heavyweight boxer which is quite uncharacteristic of the usual tall slimmer Jamaican builds. Andre only wears white boxer shorts and no mask. Patients are asked to wear masks but not required to do so. Ron has not taken his off. COVID patients have difficulty breathing and most are on oxygen support, so a mask often contributes to lowering oxygen intake which is damaging to a COVID patient, hence the lack of mask enforcement in the ward.

Every breath Andre takes is loud and strained. He, like most in this ward, are severe COVID-19 cases with their vitals at life threatening levels. The COVID hive within Andre's chest is big and without medical support his heart would just stop with exhaustion! Andre has critically low blood oxygen levels around 60 and that is with oxygen support. Ron's blood oxygen levels are normal at 97. Andre's heart rate is elevated indicating it is working overtime to pump blood oxygen to the body. Andre's total cholesterol is 386 well above the 200 maximum for normal. Ron is surprised that his 196 total cholesterol is lower than his at home readings. Ron has not eaten for 21 hours now which can contribute to lower readings.

Andre is constantly restless and agitated. The lack of blood oxygen (hypoxia) to the brain can trigger many uncharacteristic behaviors. The normal Andre is neither restless nor agitated. COVID-19 primarily attacks the lungs restricting oxygen intake and causes shortness of breath and the brain reacts like a drowning victim who cannot breathe. Panic takes over and all reason is lost. Andre has many bouts with panic and flails about dislodging his many body attached tubes and wires. Nurse Bonnie checks Andre and finds many unattached, only a nurse, not nurse technicians can reattach support tubes and wires.

## More Monitors

Bonnie goes about reattaching Andre's wires and hoses while Anna takes Ron's vitals. A knock at the door and Bonnie greets a tech delivering more monitoring gear. The doctors ordered a portable ECG heart monitor for Ron to wear. Bonnie returning to Ron's bedside announces, "I need to attach this ECG monitor to your chest, unbutton your shirt please" Ron unbuttons his shirt to expose his hairy chest. Bonnie places the five stick-on electrode patches on Ron's chest. Ron protests, "Don't you need to shave me first?" Nurse Bonnie replies, "No honey, they will be just fine on top of the hair." Bonnie attaches the five wire leads coming from the monitor to the patches on his chest. Bonnie requests, "button up your shirt." Ron buttons his shirt which neatly covers all the wires. Bonnie turns on the monitor then places it into Ron's shirt pocket. Bonnie, "All set... do you need anything?" Ron replies, "A clean bill of health and three steps to the front door please!" Ron's health to date has been exceptionally good with no hospitalizations since his military service days.

Another knock on the door… Bonnie answers and a tech hands her some items. Bonnie returns to Ron's bedside and indicates, "The doctor prescribed you some blood pressure medication. Can I give it to you in the stomach? Ron replies, "I don't normally have high blood pressure, nor do I take medication for it!" Bonnie answers, "You can refuse it… is that what you want to do?" Ron, "Yes, I'm just stressed over being here and I can self-manage my stress!" Bonnie replies, "Okay, give us a buzz if you need anything." Bonnie walks to the door and removes her protective gear, except the primary mask and places them into a bin inside the room and exits.

Ron realizes this recent heart monitor and medication activity stem from his most recent vitals spiking on heart rate and blood pressure. The stress of the move into a COVID ward has sent Ron onto a panic and he knows this is counterproductive. Ron completed some transcendental meditation classes in his early twenties. He found this discipline extremely helpful over the years in coping with life's stresses. Ron begins to meditate… Andre continues to flail and vocalize his discomfort which is not the ideal environment for quiet meditation. Ron continues to meditate for twenty minutes and emerges feeling refreshed.

## Dinner Bell

It is now 5:31 pm and a hospital worker opens the door while remaining outside and says, "Andre, you haven't ordered dinner yet, do you need help?" Andre responds, "I want the same chicken dinner I had yesterday." The voice replies, "ok, I'll place your order." Voice from outside again, "Ron, you are on water only diet so we can't order you anything… sorry!" Ron replies, "Yippie, thanks!" Meal orders in this hospital are placed by each patient from a menu specifically designed for a patient type. Andre must order from a diabetic menu. Bonnie already informed Ron of his limited diet and instructed him to only sip water and that his saline drip will supplement the water his body needs. Ron is surprised that he does not feel hungry. He last ate a big meal on New Year's Eve, 24 hours ago.

Ron adjusts the bed back to a sitting position and turns his attention to the CPAP machine sitting next to his bed. CPAP's are used by people who have difficulty sleeping due to obstructive breathing and Ron was diagnosed as such over 20 years ago. This CPAP sits atop a sturdy table on wheels. Ron rotates it around to look at it from all angles. Looking at the back of the machine he notices it has a large HEPA filter. It dawns on him… this is a big air filtering machine! Ron decides he is going to wear the CPAP  24/7 while in this ward thereby providing him with filtered air to breath. He turns the machine on and affixes the large cup mask to his face. Ron uses a less bulky mask at home but is familiar with this older style cup mask. The mask shape resembles that of a male athletic support cup, and it covers the nose and mouth. The next fifteen minutes he spends adjusting the many Velcro straps that wrap around the head to hold the mask against the face without leaking.

Andre's food arrives, he is a chow hound and there are few things he likes more than food. Jamal places the tray of food on Andre's rolling table. Andre says, "I didn't get my pudding." Jamal replies, "call the cafeteria…" and points to a whiteboard with the cafeteria phone number. The cafeteria delivery personnel do not suit up when entering the room but are double masked and trained to get in and out quickly with only two responses. 'Call your nurse.' or 'Call the cafeteria.'

Andre loudly slurps his food down which is uncharacteristic for him. The simple activity of eating tires him out. With each mouthful he gasps for air and chokes often with the stressed breathing. Ron lays in silence sympathetically listening to Andre's struggle and dreading himself getting to that stage of the disease. Ron feels his stress level climbing again and begins a short meditation to head off the anxiety.

## Distress Call

Andre climbs back into bed breathing like he just completed a marathon race. He begins loudly calling, "Nurse… Nurse!" but his voice trails off to a whisper as he is now too tired to call out. Ron is in a panic over Andre's distress calls and pushes the service call button. Five minutes pass… ten minutes pass… and still no response from the call button. Andre still sounds like he is taking his last breaths. Each patient also has a phone and Ron notices that the room whiteboard has a nurse's station phone number. Ron calls the nurses station and reports that his roommate is in distress. Another five minutes, still no hospital response.

A full twenty minutes after Ron first pushed the call button, nurse tech Maya enters the room suited up. Ron says, "he needs help!" Maya assesses Andre's condition and exclaims, "You have again pulled all your support lines off, I need to get the nurse!" Maya exits, and another four minutes pass then nurse Eleanor (Nora) enters the room. Nora finds that Andre has not just pulled his oxygen from his face, he also pulled the hose from the wall. Nora instructs Maya to get a new hose as this one is broken. Andre is now delirious from lack of oxygen. Andre also pulled the IV port from his arm, but Nora cannot reattach it while Andre is in such an agitated state, he is a big thrashing man.

Nora pulls the curtain separating the roommates to give more privacy to the activities. Ron, laying helpless is numbed by the intensity of the trauma within the room and again dreads the thought of facing a similar degrading battle with COVID. Maya returns with a new oxygen hose and a male technician Sanjay to help manage Andre and his flailing about. The disconnected oxygen is Andre's worst issue as his brain and body are being deprived of vital oxygen. Brain function is completely unpredictable when deprived of oxygen. Andre's delirium is preventing his otherwise normal reasoning in knowing that he is hurting himself. The oxygen supply is reestablished, and the trio now attempt to calm Andre down. Within three minutes Andre is no longer combative so nurse Nora begins the reattachment of his IV port. Sanjay leaves as he was called to assist from another floor. Ron deliberates, "If ever there was a man hanging on the ragged edge of life, Andre is that man!" Ron tries more meditation to clear the recent terror from his thoughts.

## Call it A Day

Nora prepares to depart the room and looks in on Ron, "Are you okay honey?" Ron replies, "Physically yes, but mentally no." Nora asks, "What is your gallbladder pain level currently?" Ron must stop and think a bit as the resent turmoil provided a distraction from his pain. Ron replies with, "Eight!" Nora indicates that the doctor already approved pain medication as needed. Ron quickly replies, "Yes please!" Nora indicates there are three to chose from and recites them. Morphine is on the list and Ron has heard of this old drug but never tried it. So, Ron replies, "Morphine." Nora responds with, "Good choice!" and leaves the room warning Andre not to pull out his support lines again.

Nora returns with the morphine and injects it into Ron's arm. Ron indicates he needs to urinate. Nora points to a tall, handled bottle hanging from the bed side rail and indicates, "Use that and go slow getting out of bed… be careful not to pull out any of your support lines like Andre over there." Nora leaves and Ron relieves himself. Ron had difficulty removing the CPAP mask which is necessary for him to stand next to the bed. The mask release catch is difficult to unclasp and the mask cannot be removed simply by ripping if off. Ron familiarizes himself with the overly complicated clasp while it is off his head. Task completed; Ron refits the mask to his face.

Thanks to the morphine Ron's pain level is down to a three so he lowers the bed into a comfortable position conducive to sleep. Closing his eyes results in cloud like images slowly moving about. Mentally exhausted, he quickly drifts into a slumber. Sleep does not last long here. Ron and Andre are awakened three more times during the night for vitals checks.

# Chapter Two:  Deep Inside the House of COVID

Day-two of Ron's hospital visit begins with the 5:00 am rounds of the hospital staff checking vitals and prepping for the 6:00 am shift change. Most of the hospital support staff are scheduled for one of two shift types, 8-hour or 12-hour shifts. The 6:00 am shift change is the only daily change where the two shifts change at the same time. The COVID hive is buzzing as the staff prepares for the shift transition, confirming their duties are complete and rooms in order before shift turnover.

As the staff come and go in the room Ron is embarrassed. Andre has constant unapologetic loud flatulence that subsequently fills the room with a foul stench. Andre is lucky in that he has lost his sense of smell, a side effect of the medication he receives for COVID. The room always has a stench... Ron wonders if the smell is also that of COVID? Andre is also given a medication once a day that produces a strong unpleasant odor in the room. Ron ponders, does the stench contribute to the continued delay in obtaining room service?

Andre asks, "When is breakfast?" Nurse technician Neshia responds, "The cafeteria opens at 6:30 but you can place your order any time after 6:00." Andre moans, "I'm hungry... and I needs some water." Ron checks his, "I need some too please." Neshia responds, "I will bring you some on my return trip." A half hour passes and still no water, Andre loudly vocalizes his need for water and becomes agitated. Moments later, Andre again loudly voices his displeasure with the service, "This place is a joke!" It will take an hour and a half for Andre to get his water. But Ron's is forgotten and is two hours before he is brought water.

The room door opens, and a voice calls from outside, Andre, "You haven't ordered breakfast yet, can I order you something?" Andre fights his brain fog and limited ability to vocalize between gasps and orders breakfast. He orders an omelet, ham-n-cheese, with home fries but is denied the home fries as they are not on his diabetic menu. Reluctantly he settles for a fruit cup and orange juice. Ron is still on a water only diet so no breakfast for him. He has not eaten in 36 hours. Ron being somewhat of a chow hound himself is surprised at his lack of appetite and suspects they are giving him appetite suppressants.

Breakfast arrives for Andre and he noisily digs in, all while voicing his displeasure with the quality and quantity of the food provided. The smell of food increases Ron's desire for something to eat. He turns his attention to Andre's TV which blares nonstop day and night. The news reports that the U.S. just surpassed twenty million reported COVID-19 cases. Ron ponders, "Was it I that pushed that number over the milestone?" The news is depressing so Ron tunes out the TV chatter.

## Disgusting Embarrassment

Andre finished his breakfast forty-five minutes ago and is beginning to thrash about in his bed. He again begins to loudly call out for a nurse but the COVID hive within his chest saps his strength to vocalize anything for long. Ron sensing Andre's heightened distress asks, "Andre, what's up?" Andre indicates he needs to go to the bathroom. Ron presses the service call button. Twenty minutes pass and no response from the service request. Ron thinks, "What a useless button!" and picks up the phone and calls the nurses station and reports that his roommate needs help going to the restroom.

Six minutes pass and still no help… Ron can hear Andre trying to get out of bed… Andre has once again torn out all his support lines and stumbles to the in-room restroom. A loud commotion begins in the restroom. Andre is banging about expelling many expletives. Ron again phones the nurses station and demands someone needs to come now and assist Andre. Nurse assistant Aditi attempts to enter the room, but Andre left the bathroom door open and it prevents the room door from opening. Several pushes and the room door opens. Aditi now inside gasps, "oh!" and yells into the hall, "Stat… Stat!" and returns to help Andre.

Andre did not make it to the toilet and is now on the restroom floor covered in his own diarrhea. The room fills with the foulest of odors. A bewildered Ron utters, "Can this get any worse?" But he knows it can as that could easily be himself soon battling COVID. They take Andre away to clean him up as there is no in room shower. This is not Andre's fault… he cannot travel to the bathroom without a nurse first disconnecting him properly. Ron concludes, "This type of debacle could be avoided with better attention to the service requests, perhaps it is a lack of staff covering the ward."

A cleaning crew enters the room, "disgusting!" is their response. It takes two people twenty minutes to clean the bathroom. Meanwhile a cleaned-up Andre returns and is in extreme respiratory distress resulting from his physical exertion and being without supplemental oxygen for thirty-five minutes. The nurses work to reattach his oxygen and other support lines. Nurse Trina begins to admonish Andre for pulling out his support lines, but Andre launches a strained objection; "I called… and called… no one came! I gots… to get out of dis place!"

The cleaning crew is done but the room still reeks. Ron asks Trina if they have any Lysol and Trina indicates she will check. None ever comes…

## Surgeon Please

Dr. Martinez, general surgeon appears at Ron's bedside, it is 10:14 am. He introduces himself as the surgeon assigned to Ron's case. He surmises, "I see you were diagnosed as having an infected gallbladder. We will need to drain the gallbladder and wait a few weeks for the infection to clear. But I see you also have COVID-19." Ron objects, "I tested negative and then positive 3 hours later! I think the second test was a false positive!" Dr. Martinez replies, "Well you are now exposed in a COVID ward and I have to proceed as if you have COVID-19." Ron pleads for another test, but Dr. Martinez reiterates, "Another test resulting in negative will not change anything that I do for you. You are exposed to COVID and likely in an incubation stage for which a test would return a false negative for three to five days." Ron groans, "God… well then what next?"

Dr. Martinez pauses in thought… "The next step is to drain the gallbladder of the infection and that procedure requires an anesthetic, but if you have COVID the anesthetic could cause respiratory complications during surgery. I need to order two different chest scans to identify any respiratory damage you may already have stemming from COVID-19. If you are clear, I can operate and place the drain. If not clear, you will need to recover form COVID before we can operate… let us get you scheduled." Andre interrupts, "Hey doc, when can I get out of here? Dr Martinez replies, "You will need to speak with the general physician, I am a surgical doctor and have no say in your release."

Ron jumps in, "Okay doc, can these tests be done today?" Doc, "depends on the availability of the lab, your nurse will let you know more." Dr. Martinez leaves Ron to ponder the added need for testing that ultimately points to a longer hospital stay. Ron sighs; "Andre, I'm screwed… I gots to get out of this place too!"

The morning activities push Ron deeper into despair as he assesses the increased certainty of catching COVID-19. He slows his breathing… while thinking about breathing in the same air that Andre is exhaling. More shivers… the despair gives way to bewildered thoughts of, will I ever see Patty, my family, or my friends again? After all, the COVID ward does not permit visitors. Phone signal strength is insufficient for phone calls and texting takes several tries. Ron utters, "When will I wake from this nightmare?" He closes his eyes and withdraws to the depths of despair.


## New COVID-19 Medication

Nurse Trina hangs a new IV bag for Andre filled with his dose of COVID medication. At this time, the only antiviral drug FDA approved for emergency use to treat COVID-19 is Veklury (Remdesivir). The administration of Remdesivir requires a 5-day hospital stay as it is only approved for intravenous slow drip use administered five times once a day. Today is Andre's fifth and final dose of Remdesivir.

Ron asks nurse Trina, "Does my IV contain Remdesivir?" Trina replies, "It does not, the doctor has not prescribed it." Ron objects, "They say I have COVID, shouldn't they be treating me for COVID?" Trina responds, "That is a conversation you need to have with your assigned general physician." Ron, "How do I obtain audience with said doctor?" Trina, "He makes rounds once a day visiting each patient." Ron, "Another process around here that could be improved upon!"

Ron looks at his phone, Patty left a text message asking how he is doing. Ron pauses… "How am I really doing?" The gallbladder pain is less… thanks to the antibiotics which now seems pale in comparison to the helpless despair of living in a deadly COVID nest. Ron sends Patty a clinical update on his condition.

## Taking a closer look

Saturday 1:45 pm, nurse Trina enters the room with a hospital gown for Ron, he is still in street clothes. Nurse Trina, "Put this on… you have a 2 o'clock appointment with the imaging lab." Ron asks, "Opening in the back?" Trina, "Yes, and transport should be here in a few minutes." Trina disconnects Ron's IV lines and heart monitor.

Lamonte arrives pushing a hospital bed. Ron remarks, "Is a bed necessary?" Lamonte, "That's what they ordered." Ron climbs aboard while trying not to flash everyone. Ron now secure Lamonte states, "We are heading to the Imaging Lab, right?" Ron replies, "No, please take me to the nearest bus terminal… I need out of here!" Lamonte chuckles. As they leave the Infectious Disease ward Ron has a feeling of release leaving COVID behind and takes a deep breath.

Entering the Imaging Lab Ron states, "This is not the bus station" Lamonte once again chuckles. Lamonte is directed to put Ron in lab #2. As they enter the lab Ron exclaims, "This is a spaceship, I saw it on the way to the hospital!" Lamonte is done being amused and leaves Ron alone in the room. Two exceptionally large machines occupy the very cold alien ship probing bay.

Lab Tech Clair enters the lab from an adjoining room. Ron expected the aliens to have large heads and big eyes, but this alien looks normal. Clair confirms with Ron that he is the scheduled 2 o'clock patient for a CT scan. Ron questions the expectation of the scan. Clair explains that the scan will help identify any COVID lung damage. Ron declares, "I do not have COVID!" Clair, "Well this scan will help in confirming your conviction." Ron is wheeled under the smaller machine and instructed to inhale deeply and hold the breath until told to breath. Two scans are completed in less than a minute. Ron asks, "How long before the results are back? Clair responds, "A few hours and your doctor will review the results with you."

Lamonte waited outside the room and returns to transport Ron back to the COVID ward. As they reenter the Infectious Disease ward Ron's sense of hopelessness returns and consequently, fiddles with his facemask. Upon entering the room Ron addresses Andre, "I tried to escape but they caught me!" Andre does not respond and is wearing his "I am miserable face." Nurse Trina reattaches

Ron's IV lines and heart monitor. Ron then replaces the hospital gown with his street clothes just in case he has an opportunity to run.

## Dinner in The Ward

It is 4:10 pm and the room door opens followed by a voice from outside, "Andre, you have not ordered you dinner yet. I can place the order for you if you like." Andre chooses the special, chicken pot pie and a side salad. Ron… "You are on a water only diet and I can not order you anything." Ron sighs, it has been forty-eight hours since Ron last ate New Year's Eve dinner and is beginning to feel the hunger.

While at the imaging lab Ron missed the doctor making his daily rounds. Which could have been a rare opportunity to spar with someone in charge about getting another COVID test and getting out of the Infectious Disease Ward. Ron is still COVID symptom free, while his roommate is in full blown COVID distress.

Ron, while wearing his CPAP mask throughout the day, adjusts the straps for use while being awake. The mask fits loosely about his face during the day providing filtered breathing air to the nose and mouth. The loose fit also allows the mask to be pushed aside for speaking when needed. Otherwise, communication is near impossible when the mask is tightly secured for nighttime sleeping.

Andre's dinner arrives with a welcome aroma covering up the foul smell of flatulence. Andre struggles to sit up to eat but food is the drug he will do anything for, so he manages. Ron tries to ignore the slurping and grunting. He wishes for the headphones from home or earplugs. Earplugs… another item to put on his request list! Andre finishes his dinner and complains, "Not enough to feed a mouse!" Andre struggles to stand next to his bed and urinates into his portable urinal bottle. Ron reflects, "Real five-star accommodations here!"


## Another Bloody Mess

Another blood cart arrives in the room pushed by blood lab technician Kaia. She informs Ron that she is here to collect some blood. Ron sighs and responds, "I have small deep veins, and everyone is having difficulty drawing my blood!" Kaia, "Let me take a look." Kaia's first attempt fails to find a vein and now searches for another location. She presses on the inner elbow joint and Ron protests, "That area is all stuck out and very sore!" Kaia finds a location lower on the arm and is successful for a moment, but the blood stops flowing almost immediately. She tries to shift the needle to reestablish the flow and after several twists Ron protests. Kaia removes the needle and without a word packs up her supplies and leaves the room. Ron mumbles, "Thank od for the two-strike rule!"

On any given day outside the hospital the private labs have trouble drawing blood from Ron. Here in the hospital Ron is dehydrated which makes drawing blood even harder than normal. He is told to only sip water and that the IV will provide the necessary fluids. The same IV that sits empty for hours because a nurse is too busy to replace it. Dehydration is not a monitored vital here in the hospital, so he suffers the painful consequences whenever blood needs to be drawn.

Forty minutes pass and another blood cart arrives pushed by Alisha. She informs Ron that she is here to collect blood samples. Ron sighs, "Again already! Someone just tried unsuccessfully. I am a difficult stick. I have bruises all up and down my arms. Everyone is having difficulty drawing my blood!" Alisha responds with a, "Humm" and inspects Ron's arm full of bruises. Alisha, "I see you are receiving a blood thinner in your IV in prep for a gallbladder procedure. The thinner enhances the occurrence of bruising when blood is taken." Alisha searches for a sight to draw blood. Alisha's first attempt is successful in drawing two tubes of blood. Ron is relieved, "Can I request you for all future tests?" Alisha replies, "We obtain our next assignment from a computer which uses our current location and the proximity to a patient needing blood work." Ron replies, "Well stay nearby… good job and thank you!"

## Bedtime Hallucinations

It is only 9 pm on Saturday but Ron feels exhausted. Not physically exhausted but mentally drained and prepares for sleep. He begins by tightening the CPAP mask straps that hold the mask in place. The mask must be secured airtight to help prevent sleep apnea. Ron uses a CPAP to relieve the side effects of obstructive apnea, which means he stops breathing and snores heavily while sleeping. The bed controls amuse Ron as he plays with the adjustments to obtain the perfect sleeping position. Now for some more sleeping with COVID!

Moments later Andre begins calling out, "Nurse… nurse…" Ron presses the bedside call button. The nurses station responds quicker this time, "Can I help you?" Ron replies, "My roommate is calling out for help please hurry!" Nurses tech Maya enters the room, "Who needs help?" Andre replies, "I needs to go to the bathroom!" Maya disconnects Andre from his IV and oxygen hoses and he is off to the in-room toilet.

Maya asks Ron if he is ok. Ron responds, "Can I get some pain medication to sleep better? Maya, "I will check with the nurse." Andre returns and Maya reconnects him. Nurse Eleanor (Nora) enters the room with morphine for Ron. Nora asks, "Did the morphine work ok for you last night?" Ron, "Yes thanks." Nora administers the medication.

Ron did not bring a phone charger to the hospital and his phone battery is nearly drained. He asks Nora, "Does the hospital have a charging station for phones?" Nora replies, "Not officially but there are a number of chargers in the family visiting room, which is not used since COVID." Ron asks, "Would you mind trying to plug my phone into one? I do not need it the rest of the evening." Nora agrees and takes his phone.

Ron closes his eyes… within minutes slow moving cloud-like patterns ebb and flow across his eyelids. Like looking at puffy clouds… shapes appear, then progressively vivid colors add more interest. Eventually full lifelike images morph from one to another, no frightening images like sleeping with COVID. The stress of the day is forgotten thanks to this drug induced ocular dance…

# Chapter three:  Change Is Coming

Sunday, day-three of Ron's hospital visit begins with the 5:00 am rounds of the hospital staff checking vitals and prepping for the 6:00 am shift change. Once again nurse tech Maya finds Andre's IV line disconnected, she goes about reconnecting him. Andre asks, "When can I get out of here… I needs to get out of here?" Maya answers. "That will be for your doctor to approve."

Most COVID patients are admitted to the hospital because they have severe respiratory complications that qualify them to receive the Remdesivir drug. Most patients stay between nine and ten days giving the Remdesivir time to do some good. Andre completed his five-day Remdesivir dose yesterday and is on day six of his hospital stay. Andre's breathing is still labored and requires around the clock supplemental oxygen. Without the supplemental oxygen Andre falls into a lack of oxygen delirium.

Ron is surprised at how well he slept and gives thanks to the morphine but is disappointed in that, all this was not just a bad dream. Adjusting the bed back Ron sits up and loosens the CPAP mask for daytime use. The air in the room remains heavy with the usual stench, which startles Ron into pushing the mask back to his face. Ron just realized that the air filter on the CPAP also provides some relief from smells. He also realizes that he would most likely tolerate a COVID ventilator better than most people as a CPAP is similar but with a much less aggressive delivery system.

Maya is finished reattaching Andre then turns to ask Ron if he is okay? Ron explains that his phone is on a charger in the Family Visiting Room and asks if she or someone could return it when possible. Maya suggests a call to the Nurses Station and make the same request as she has other rooms to service first. It takes Ron several calls and repeated explanation of the need but eventually Ron's fully charged phone is returned by late-morning.


## Get Out of Here

Andre asks everyone who enters the room, "When can I get out of here?" Even the breakfast delivery person. Nurse Trina enters the room, "Andre, you are being evaluated for release today. You must have a place to quarantine and you must have oxygen equipment at that location. Someone will call you to arrange for equipment delivery." The damage in Andre's lungs is severe. He will not survive COVID recovery without ongoing supplemental oxygen. His girlfriend offered to be his caregiver during home recovery and will have her hands full. Ron doubts she will last more than a day with his off and on delirium, which occurs often when he refuses to wear the supplemental oxygen.

Ron ponders his own discharge, should it happen. Going back to staying with Patty is not an option as it would risk exposing her to COVID. He deems Andre a lucky man in that he has a place to go and recover. He also delights in the thought of Andre leaving, not for a personal dislike. It is more the witnessing of Andre's agony which serves as an alarming reminder of what Ron must look forward to as COVID develops in his lungs! How could it not... day and night he is breathing the expelled air from a seriously infected patient! Ron slips into a deeper depression over this new dilemma and mumbles, "I sure fell into a deep dark hole this time!"

Maya enters the room, "Andre, put this gown on… you need to demonstrate that you are ambulatory before you are released. Andre, "What?" Maya responds, "We are going for a walk." Maya disconnects Andre and he gets dressed. Maya and Andre walk to the end of the hall and back. Maya checks Andre's heart rate and oxygen levels and records them. Andre's oxygen is reattached but not his IV. Winded, he lays down and labors to breath.

Andre's bedside phone rings… he is not answering the phone. Ron calls out, "Andre, you need to answer the phone." Andre in a labored voice, "Where is it?" Ron, "On the stand next to your bed." Andre answers the phone… his recent walk put him into a fog and now the phone conversation with hospital administration staff is difficult. After some persistence, data is gathered, and the arrangements are completed for Andre's release. Andre hangs up the phone and announces, "I'm getting out-a here!" Ron, "That is great news Andre, have a speedy recovery!"

## Hearing Voices

The door opens and a mysterious voice from the other side asks, "Andre, do you want to order lunch?" Andre places his order topped with cookies and chocolate pudding. He is denied the desserts due to his diabetic diet. Andre replies, "I'm getting out-a here and needs to celebrate." Still denied he settles for diet jell-O. The far-side voice returns, "Ron, you can have chicken or beef broth if you like?" Ron, "Chicken, thanks." It's been sixty-five hours since Ron last ate solid food so at this point even broth sounds appetizing.

The noon news blares on the TV… more depressing statistics on the COVID death rate. Ron is still COVID symptom free but most likely in the incubation stage, which often does not present symptoms. This is the period when the COVID virus silently builds its hive within the lungs of the clueless host.

Lunch arrives, Ron's tray includes a small cup size covered bowl with a side of salt and pepper packets. A taste test reveals a disappointing, cold, and weak broth. Regardless, the cup is quickly emptied. Ron sighs, "Everything about this place is depressing!" Andre quickly cleans his plate and remarks, "I cannot wait to eat some good food again!" Ron replies, "I cannot wait to just eat food again!" Ron asks, "What is your favorite food?" Andre responds, "One of my favorites… my woman is making me Jerk chicken tonight for dinner." Ron, "Sounds good! I'm easy, pizza does it for me."

The vitals cart returns to the room and the tech heralds, "Andre, one last check of your vitals please." The check reveals that Andre's oxygen levels are low and blood pressure is high. Ron's vitals are checked, and all are within normal range. Suddenly Andre makes a dash to the bathroom, which only requires removing his oxygen mask. He is no longer attached to an IV, so the dash is without peril this time. Ron looks at the TV, it is still projecting fear to the public over the COVID virus. Ron grumbles, "As soon as he leaves, I'm going to turn that crap off… Two less depressing things in this room!"

## Can You Help Me Doc

The surgeon, Doctor Martinez enters the room and addresses Ron, "I looked at your CT scan and do not see anything concerning in your chest. I am scheduling you for a nuclear scan. This will give me a good look at the gallbladder and a better assessment of the infection surrounding it." Ron huffs, "Well, if there is no indication of COVID in my lungs… that means I can get out of this ward, right?" Martinez replies, "That is not my call, you need to speak with the general physician." Ron huffs again, "Everything around here is someone else's job, but everyone seems to be working hard at keeping me in this ward. You are the only physician talking to me. I requested audience with the general physician and was told… paraphrasing, he wanders about the floor and I need to wait until he wanders into my room! I am really stressed out here, can you help me doc?" Martinez sighs, "I hear your concern and will send your general physician a message to speak with you. Let's get that next scan going so we can address the gallbladder."

A few minutes later… Maya enters the room, "Ron you are scheduled for another scan, put this gown on please." Maya disconnects Ron's IV and heart monitor. Feeling freed, Ron contemplates running for the door! But Jackson from transport arrives with a hospital bed and blocks the door. Ron walks into the hallway and climbs aboard, "Wee, off we go… at least I get out of the ward for a while!" The world feels lighter exiting the locked doors of the Infectious Disease Ward. A rare grin appears…

Ron is wheeled into imaging lab #2 again. Clair is waiting and instructs Jackson to, "Park him next to the nuclear scanner." Pointing to the larger machine in the room. Clair instructs Ron to lay on the bench attached to the scanner. Clair then explains the nuclear scanning process, "This will only take a few minutes. Jackson, stick around please. You may feel some pressure as the radioactive dye is injected. The injection takes about eight seconds and the subsequent 2 scans run about fifteen seconds each. Please remain still during the scanning procedures."

Clair begins to connect the radioactive dye injection tube to the port already in Ron's arm. Having some difficulty making the connection Clair looks closer and remarks, "This looks to be an 20-gauge port, which is too small. You will need an 18-gauge port to handle the volume during the rapid injection. You need to return to your room and have someone insert a larger port." Ron objects, "Can the port be put in here, sounds simple?" Clair, "No, we do not have a qualified specialist in this lab. Also, larger ports mean inserting larger needles requiring a specialist to locate a larger vein and insert the needle deep enough into the vein to avoid rapid injection blow-out." A chill shakes Ron as he recalls the difficulty they had installing the smaller port and now a larger one is needed.

## More Stabbing Pain

Back in his room Ron finds Andre is missing… he was released while Ron was in the Imaging Center. Ron turns off the TV and remarks, "Darn, I missed wishing him well. Hope he has a quick recovery… for his girlfriend's sake!" Trina enters the room. "Ron, I hear we need to get you another port and reading your chart notes… I see you have a reputation as a difficult stick. We need to get you back to the Imaging Lab before they close for the day so let us see how it goes." Ron groans as Trina approaches or was that a growl? Both of Trina's attempts fail in attaching a new port. Apologetic Trina says, "I will see if someone from the Blood Lab can help with this."

Luciana from the Blood Lab enters the room. She looks at Trina and motions her outside the room, "I could not pull blood from this man and you want me to put a port in? I will try if he lets me." Luciana reenters the room and makes two failed attempts to insert a port. Head nurse Emma enters the room carrying port supplies. The hour wait between sticking tries is out the window as Ron needs to return to the Imaging Center. Emma takes Ron's arm and inspects it, "Fairly bruised up!" She reaches for Ron's other arm and Trina jumps in, "This is for a nuclear test so it can not be in the same arm as the IV." Emma returns to searching the right arm and makes two failed attempts to put the port in. Trina notices that Ron is sweating, "Are you okay honey?" Ron begins to shiver… Emma remarks, "He is having a vasovagal episode, increase his saline flow!" Ron soon recovers and remarks, "That was crazy, I'm done with this for a while!" The hospital staff leaves the room.

Forty minutes pass and Blood Lab Tech Fanibhusan enters the room. Ron recognizes him from a prior visit and recalls he was good with a needle. Fanibhusan looks at the port and comments, "A smaller port would be easier to place." Trina replies, "It must be the larger port to accommodate a nuclear imaging test." Fanibhusan misses on his first attempt in the forearm. He inspects the back of the hand and wrist, "This area is not ideal for a port, but it is less torn up." Fanibhusan secures the port on the second attempt. The port is placed on the backside of Ron's wrist. Ron comments, "It really hurts to move or even use my hand with it there." Trina responds, "Well we only need this port for the test and after we can remove it. Let us see if we can get you scheduled back in the Imaging Center."

Trina returns to the room, "Ron, I was not able to get you into the Imaging Center today as it is too late in the day. They did have an opening for tomorrow, so you are scheduled for 9:00 am." Ron looks at his wrist and wiggles some fingers, "Ouch, I can not close my hand!" A voice calls into the room, "Ron, do you want some broth for dinner?" Ron, "Yes, I will try beef this time and can I get two?" Response, "No, you are on a minimal liquid diet." Ron receives most of his liquid intravenously through an IV. He reclines the bed some and closes his eyes.

## Cleanup In Room 106

A stir in the room interrupts Ron's slumber. It is Trudy, a member of the cleaning staff pulling a cleaning cart into the room. Trudy introduces herself to Ron and explains she is here to clean and prep the space that Andre occupied. Ron comments, "My ex-roommate was a very messy person." Trudy is a talkative middle-aged woman with a strong country accent and engages Ron with conversation as she goes about her cleaning tasks.

Ron asks Trudy if she had COVID yet? Trudy replies, "I don't think so but don't know for sure. I had a few bad colds last Spring which may or may not have been COVID. I've only worked here for 3 months." Ron queries, "Doesn't working in the COVID ward scare you? It sure scares the bejesus out of me being here!" Trudy responds, "No, I always wear a mask and work with cleaning products all day. Unless they force me, I won't get the vaccination and fear that more than catching the virus."

Ron is surprised, "Dang you're tough, I'm getting the vaccination when its available. I've seen the suffering it causes!" Trudy spends the better part of an hour cleaning the room and chatting nonstop. Ron enjoys the conversation, being it has been three days since he last had a normal conversation.

Dinner arrives and the cup of cool broth is consumed in a few seconds. The beef flavor is no better than the chicken, in fact, dish-soap would be equally tasty. Ron is confounded. "I do not feel famished and it has been 72 hours since I last ate solid food. That New Year's dinner was really filling!" Ron closes his eyes and takes a deep breath, "Now this is peaceful."

## New Roommate

It is 6:12pm and a commotion in the doorway interrupts Ron's slumber. He opens his eyes to find a young man in a wheelchair being pushed into the room followed by three hospital staff. Ron finds it unusual in that all three employees are men. The young man in the wheelchair is eighteen-year-old Liam. He is an autistic patient from a nearby institution and has been institutionalized most of his life.

Liam has a severe COVID infection with extremely low oxygen levels. He was brought to the hospital to receive the Remdesivir medication, which will help speed his recovery from COVID. Liam is a low functioning level-3 diagnosed autistic patient. Meaning he has extremely limited communication skills. Liam is agitated and it is quickly apparent that he is not here of his own free will. He sports a restraining jacket which further explains the three-man escort. He is wheeled to the bedside all the while loudly voicing his displeasure with what is going on. His voicing attempts do not resemble that of words, but rather a strained hysteria of gibberish.

The crew remove the restraining jacket and struggle with Liam to place him into the hospital bed. Liam repeats a sound that may be his version of 'no' over and over as they attempt to get him settled. Liam will not remain in the bed. Nurse Mary leaves the room and returns with head nurse Amanda. The nursing team attach restraints to Liam to keep him in the hospital bed. Liam is no stranger to restraints, but he still becomes increasingly agitated. Once Liam is restrained, the male members leave the room and the nursing team connect Liam to oxygen.

Nurse Mary looks in Ron's direction and walks to his bedside. She explains in a whisper that Liam is incapable of communicating orally and asks Ron to contact the Nurses Station should Liam do something that poses a danger. Ron, "How will I know? The curtain is pulled for privacy and I would like to keep it that way. I'm not comfortable being responsible for his wellbeing. Plus, the nursing staff response is dismal!" Mary replies, "That's fine, use your best judgement. No one is going to hold you responsible." Ron whispers, "Sorry, I cannot stay in this room. You will need to strap me down to keep me here!" Mary whispers back, "I will notify administration of the situation and of your discomfort." Ron, "Thank you, and would you mind placing my phone on a charger in the family visiting room?" Mary, "Sure…"

The hospital staff leave the room turning the lights off as they exit. The sudden darkness causes Liam to pause for a few seconds but quickly returns to his vocal displeasure of the situation. Ron sighs, "I did not think it possible, but I would gladly trade this new roommate for Andre's return. Hope he enjoyed his jerked chicken this evening." Ron internalizes, "In the future, should I ever feel depressed about my life sucking... I now have insight into a hell that no one should have to endure."

## Hush Baby

Liam's life on a good day is a lonely and confusing one. His current problem, lack of oxygen caused by COVID, compounds his normal confusion and now he is terrified. Andre had a normal functioning brain but suffered hysteria when deprived of oxygen, but he understood why it was happening. Liam on the other hand, can not comprehend why his already frightening world just got much worse. COVID is a wicked virus that even preys on the weak and it should not be taken lightly!

The endless crying and babble continue into the evening. Liam, not having the lung capacity to be extremely loud still manages a nonstop vocal barrage declaring his existence and discontent. It has been an hour since the hospital staff left the room and Ron is going mad listening to Liam's nonsensical narration. Knowing Liam cannot understand conversation Ron wishes he could sing, but his singing voice would just frighten Liam. Desperate to get Liam to abandon the endless chatter he tries speaking... and calls out, "Testing 1, 2, 3... Testing 1, 2, 3." Liam pauses for about 10 seconds and slowly restarts his barrage. Ron repeats the test, but this time Liam only pauses for a few seconds. One last try, "I wish I had a cookie!" No pause this time. He gives up that approach.

Sound seems to be the only option in Ron's arsenal, another idea comes to mind. The CPAP machine has differing alarms, breaking loose the face mask without first pausing the machine sounds an alarm. What the heck... Ron pulls loose the mask causing a whooshing air sound that puts Liam on pause. Then the alarm sounds causing Liam to grunt but he remains on pause. After a few seconds, Ron considers the alarm sound to be no better than listening to Liam. The alarm is silenced, Liam remains silent for another twenty seconds then slowly restarts. Ron wonders if Liam can make a connection that his voice causes the alarm and silence keeps it off. Ron restarts the alarm and Liam pauses again... good so far. The alarm is shut off but after only ten seconds Liam slowly restarts the jabber. Ron tries several more times, but Liam becomes insensitive to the alarm going off, never making the cause-and-effect connection. It is a failed experiment but counts as a distraction for Ron.

The room lights come on and vitals tech Sofia wheels a vitals cart into the room and announces to Liam that she is here to check his vitals. The lights and Sofia startle Liam causing him to pause. But Sofia's approach to his bedside result in a loud outburst. Sofia quickly steps back and comments, "Going to need help." Sofia moves to Ron and begins taking his vitals. Nurse tech Sanjay enters the room and asks, "You need help?" Sofia, "Yes, I need help with Liam over there." Sanjay approaches Liam's bedside attempting to engage him in conversation, but Liam launches another loud burst of gibberish. Sanjay responds, "I see!"

Sofia and Sanjay attempt to calm Liam with soothing slow talk but it is not effective. Liam's vocalization escalates to a burst of shouts followed by panting between each burst. It is clear to everyone in the room that he is a very unhappy young man. Head nurse Amanda enters the room, "How long has he been without an oxygen mask?" Sofia, "It was in place when I first entered the room." Sanjay responds, "He started thrashing about when I approached him, it came loose in the last few minutes." Amanda, "This is a new patient and needs to be closely monitored… surely the three of us can gather his vitals."

The hospital crew manages to collect Liam's vitals and reattach his oxygen despite his objections. Amanda instructs Mary to remain behind and try to calm Liam. Ron asks Mary, "Any word on a room change for me?" Mary replies, "I will check." Ron sighs silently, "More lip service!" Ron's head is throbbing from the intensity of the day and asks Mary for some aspirin. Same response, "I will check."

Mary is unable to calm Liam and exits the room turning out the lights. The sudden darkness causes Liam to stop vocalizing but now his breathing has a sniffling tremble. Liam is quiet for less than a minute and slowly resumes his utterances. Ron stares into the darkness, "Soo much suffering in here!" Ron is sympathetic to Liam's predicament but at the same time feels powerless to help in any meaningful fashion. Frustrated and exhausted Ron yields to the sandman.

## Liam's Song

The CPAP alarm startles Ron from his strained slumber, it is 10:40pm. The CPAP alarm cannot be disabled completely but Ron spent hours adjusting the alarm thresholds, so now the machine presents minimal alarms. The current alarm sounded due to Ron entering a severe event of not breathing for thirty seconds. Ron presses reset and the alarm shuts off. His head still hurts and wonders what happened to the request for aspirin? The alarm also put Liam on pause for half a minute. Ron tinkers with the upper bed adjustments seeking a sleeping angle that does not set off the alarm.

Liam resumes vocalizing displeasure with his predicament. Ron stares into the darkness and contemplates Liam's raucous gibberish, "Could this be the language of COVID aliens attempting to communicate?" He does not repeat the same sound over and over. There are many variants to his chanting which suggests possible meaning. The sound is eerie in that it could be words exaggerated in a long slow expression.

Ron is startled by the revelations of his own thoughts… "Liam's song! His droning on… it closely resembles that of incantations. Ron trembles, "Holy crap… this is demonic!" …The devil be damned as he pounds the drums harder inside Ron's head. Frightened and feeling claustrophobic, Ron tugs at the thick tight straps wrapped around his head which hold the CPAP mask in place. Suddenly a burst of light fills the room… Ron partially leaps from the bed, "What da holy hell?..."

# Chapter Four:  Time to Move On

The startling burst of light in the room is thanks to nurse Mary turning on the lights as she entered. Mary proclaims, "Ron, we have you another room to move into… are you ready." Ron, "Thank God, I am ready… to go crazy here! Did you happen to bring any aspirin?" Mary, "No it is not on your list of authorized medications. We can get you some morphine once you get settled." Ron looks up at the clock, "Eleven… five hours of hell!" Mary, "Sorry for the delay." …Unknowingly, Ron's delay was due to the new roommate having a bowel accident, like Andre's, requiring a lengthy room clean-up.

Mary disconnects Ron from the IV and escorts him to the hallway where Calvin from transport awaits with a wheelchair. While getting settled in the chair Ron asks, "Can you take me to the nearest back door? They are trying to kill me in here!" Calvin chuckles, "Hang in there, bro!" Ron asks Calvin, "Will we pass the Family Visiting Center? My phone is charging in there." Calvin, "You need to work with your nurse on that."

It is a short trip and Calvin announces their arrival at room 116 and locks the chair wheels. Mary approaches pushing Ron's IV stand, "Here we are… Let me introduce you to Harry your new roommate." Ron protests, "What, no single rooms available?" Mary responds, "No, not in this ward." Ron stammers, "Well then, another COVID catching opportunity it is… off we go!" Ron mumbles, "This guy cannot be any scarier than the last two?"

Ron and Harry are introduced. Harry is 84 years old, single, and recently moved from Ohio to live with his daughter and her family in New Jersey. Harry was hospitalized thirty-two days ago with COVID and completed a Remdesivir treatment over three weeks ago. His lungs were severely damaged by COVID and he is struggling with recovery. Ron bids Harry hello, but Harry can only muster a head nod in return. Harry sits in a custom wheelchair that resembles a motorized La-Z-boy recliner on wheels. Harry has limited mobility and lives and sleeps in this comfortable cushioned chair even when at home.

The extensive COVID damage to Harry's lungs is causing a severe lack of blood oxygen making him a ventilator candidate but he has, so far, refused that treatment. Harry spent most of his life battling anxiety and was diagnosed as having a panic disorder. His battle with COVID frequently triggers the panic disorder, further complicating COVID recovery. The panic attacks cause heart palpitations that sound an alarm at the nurses' station indicating he is having an event.

While Harry sits silently in a hopeless slouch, Ron winces as he takes note of the anguished fear carved into Harry's face. Ron compares Andre's more energetic battle with that of Harry's and this is what the battle looks like when the energy to fight is depleted. The relentless suffering caused by COVID is intense, exhausting and depressing. Harry is visibly worn out from the fight.


## Day is Done

Mary reconnects Ron to his IV and checks the heart monitor connections. Ron asks, "Where is my CPAP machine?" Mary indicates, "The machine can only be moved by a Sleep Lab tech, and a tech will move it shortly." Mary asks, "Do you still need pain medication?" Ron, "Yes, more than ever thanks!" Mary, "Okay, I will be back shortly with that."

Harry and Ron are alone now, and it is almost midnight. Harry tries to speak but no distinguishable words come out. Ron looks at Harry, "This all sucks the big one Harry!" Harry nods in agreement. Harry's TV is on and also runs day and night, it is a necessary distraction for him. Laying in a hospital bed for many days it becomes easy to lose the day or night perspective.

The CPAP machine is wheeled into the room by Sleep Lab tech Marjorie. She looks at Ron, "Is this yours?" Ron responds, "Yes, can you put it on my left side please?" Marjorie, "It needs to go on your right side unless you are not using the oxygen connection." Ron, "Right, I am not using the oxygen." Marjorie plugs in the CPAP and powers it up, "Are you having any problems with the machine?" Ron, "Not really, but it occasionally sounds an E3 alarm when I have a severe event." Marjorie, "Let's take a look… These settings are all messed up!" Ron, "Since I'm not using oxygen there is only one setting when in CPAP mode and that is my pressure which is eleven." Marjorie, "No, the alarm settings are not set correctly." Ron, "I would like to turn all the alarms off but that is not an option with this machine. I spent over two hours downloading the manual and adjusting the settings so that the machine presents minimal alarms now." Marjorie, "You are not permitted to make any adjustments to this machine! You may press the power on or off only. I need to reset the settings." Ron protests, "The alarms wake me every few minutes if they are set in a normal range!" Marjorie ignores Ron and resets the alarm settings and leaves.

Mary entered the room with Ron's morphine and was waiting for Marjorie to finish. Mary asks, "What is your gallbladder pain level?" Ron, "Right now my headache pain well exceeds the gallbladder pain. The bladder pain is maybe a six and the head is a solid ten!" Mary administers the medication and asks, "Do you want the lights on or off?" Ron responds, 'Off…' Harry does not reply. The light from the TV is sufficient as a night light.

## Alarming Times

Adjusting the bed and pulling the covers up, Ron prepares for sleep. Taking a deep breath and staring at the swirling ceiling the headache relents to the morphine. The quiet of the room calms Ron's soul. The mild hallucinations provide a visual lullaby and transport Ron into a deep sleep.

At 1:48am a blaring alarm startles Ron from his deep sleep! It takes awhile for Ron to regain enough consciousness to assess the situation. The CPAP alarm sounded… Ron presses the silence button and reprimands himself for touching a button not deemed authorized by tech Marjorie. Exhausted, Ron closes his eyes and quickly falls asleep, but not for long. The CPAP alarm sounds again only minutes later. After a third such alarm Ron presses the service button at his bedside.

With a fourth alarm now sounding a service response comes, "Do you need help?" Ron, "Yes, my CPAP keeps throwing an alarm!" The voice returns, "I will notify the Sleep Lab for you." The alarm sounds several more times, but Ron grows weary of the repeated annoyance and refuses to press the silence button any longer. Harry is stirring but silent.

Forty-five minutes later Marjorie enters the room and proclaims, "You know you can silence the alarm?" Ron responds, "That is not a button you authorized me to touch! Besides, it does not remain silenced." Marjorie makes some on-screen adjustments to the alarms and asks Ron to give that a try. Ron asks, "Are you going to hang around?" Marjorie, "I will hang at the nurses' station for a few." Ron sighs and lays back.

Less than a minute passes and the alarm sounds again. Ron presses the service button and Marjorie enters the room moments later. Once again, she makes on-screen adjustments and leaves the room. Same scenario occurs… Marjorie, "I do not think this will work for you." Ron, "It worked the past two nights. I had the settings near perfect for me, but you insisted on changing them!" Marjorie, "Perhaps we can bring you another machine tomorrow." Ron, "Perhaps you can bring someone that knows what they are doing!" Marjorie leaves in a huff…

A few minutes later Mary enters the room, "What are we going to do? I understand you broke your CPAP!" Ron, "Is that what she told you? It worked fine until she messed with it, I didn't touch it today!" Mary, "Can you sleep without it tonight?" Ron, "I really do not want to, my apnea is severe. I might be able to fix the settings but was told not to touch the settings." Mary, "Right, I was also told you cannot touch the settings, but I am not going to sit here and watch you all night." Mary grins and leaves the room. Ron pulls the CPAP screen to his bedside and using the manual begins recalibrating the alarms. A few more alarms sound during the night but a few are more tolerable than many.


## Foggy Morning

It is 4:15 a.m. Monday and Elisa enters the room pushing a vitals cart. The room lights waken both Harry and Ron. Ron still in a drug induced fog, "Good God… I spend day and night in bed but get no sleep!" Elisa apologizes and takes Ron's vitals which are normal. Harry on the other hand has a low oxygen level of 57 and low heart rate of 47 bpm and an above normal body temperature. Ron quickly returns to sleep and Harry flips thru the TV channels.

Another alarm sounds, Ron opens one squinting eye in Harry's direction hoping that it is Harry's alarm this time. nope, it is Ron's IV indicating that a bag change is needed. Ron presses the service button and mumbles, "I can't take any more of this and my COVID hasn't even kicked in yet!" A voice calls out, "Can I help you?" Ron, "Yes, I need an IV bag change." Voice, "Okay, will be in shortly." Mary silences the alarm and replaces Ron's IV bag. Ron asks, "My phone is on a charger in the Family Visiting Center, can someone bring it to me?" Mary, "I will check." Mary returns a few minutes later with Ron's phone. Ron thanks Mary and asks, "Do you have a quiet broom closet that I can curl up in?" Mary replies with a smile, "Well stop calling me and things will be quiet!" Tired, Ron drifts off immediately despite Harry's TV channel surfing.

Room lights again, it is the morning room check prior to the 6 am shift change. Ron squints, "Can I get some more water?" Mary, "Sure, Harry… are you okay?" Harry stammers but fails to produce words, and in frustration, points to his full catheter bag. Mary empties his bag, snugs the covers and gives him a shoulder pat. Ron asks, "Will I be able to order breakfast today? It's been four days since I last ate." Mary replies, "Your chart still indicates a liquid diet. Please discuss that with your doctor when you see him today." Ron, "He is avoiding me… and my questions as to why I am in a COVID ward!"  Still tired, Ron secures the CPAP mask and lays back while thinking, "Andre, I absolutely gots to get out of dis place too!"

Harry's breakfast arrives at seven fifteen. Ron stirs from the noise and to a greater extent the smell of food. While looking at his bedside table he notices a juice box on the table. Looking closer it is a Very Berry sugar free juice box. Ron hates the bitter taste of diet anything but manages to slurp the last drop, but quickly regrets his action, "Ugh, that dreadful taste is going to remain in my mouth all morning." Harry has scrambled eggs and a fruit cup. He is too depressed to eat and pushes the food about his plate.

## Silent Prayer

Ron attempts a conversation with Harry, but Harry becomes frustrated trying to muster speech. Ron lays back in silent prayer, "God he is in bad shape!" Harry then starts whacking his plate with a spork. Ron can now see the anguish in Harry's face and places a call to the nurses' station, "My roommate is having an episode of some sort… please send someone!"

It takes six minutes for someone to respond to the help request. Nurse tech Cassa enters the room and asks, "Someone need help?" Ron looks at Harry who has his breakfast scattered about and gasping for air. Cassa asks,

"What is the problem honey?" Cassa presses the call button and begins to check Harry's vitals. Harry is having another panic attack. The nurses' station replies and Cassa requests Harry's medication. A few minutes pass and Nurse Bonnie enters the room with the medication which is administered into Harry's stomach area. It takes a few minutes for the medicine to calm Harry and in the meantime Cassa cleans up his scattered breakfast.

Harry and his family have not seen each other since he arrived 33 days ago due to the hospital, 'no visitor policy.' In the past two weeks he managed a few short text messages to his daughter. She calls the room phone, but Harry rarely answers and if he does it is difficult for him to form words and abruptly hangs up in tears. His daughter frantically calls back the hospital in tears begging for an update on her father's condition.

Ron stares at the ceiling, "Hospitals are so depressing… I could not work here… it would break me mentally… God bless the people that do this work!" Ron's thoughts are interrupted by sleep lab tech Tim who is pushing a CPAP cart. Looking at Ron's CPAP he asks, "You need a CPAP replaced?" Ron replies, "Unless the replacement has no alarms, I doubt a replacement will help me. Can I use my personal CPAP in place of this one?" Tim replies, "Sure, many people bring in their home machines." Ron, "Then I'm going to try and get my machine here." Tim, "Okay, I will return this one." Ron gathers up his phone and sends Patty a text asking if she would be okay with delivering his CPAP to the front desk.

## Scheduled Test

Nurse tech Cassa enters the room with a hospital gown in hand and hands it to Ron, "Put this on you have a 9:00 am appointment at the Imaging Lab. Transport will be here soon." Cassa detaches Ron's IV and heart monitor. Ron asks, "I need to urinate, can I use the bathroom since I am unhooked?" Cassa, "Certainly, be careful walking." Ron grabs the gown to change in the bathroom.

Lamonte from transport arrives with a wheelchair and greets Ron, "They had the wrong room on the transport order." Ron, "Oh, they moved me here late last night." Lamonte, "We got you now!" Lamonte seats Ron in the chair and wheels him to the Imaging Lab. Lamonte is asked to wait as the scan will not take long.

Imaging tech Clair confirms Ron as the patient by scanning his wristband and a few questions. Clair announces, "It says here we have you scheduled for a hepatobiliary nuclear scan of the gallbladder and kidney, right?" Ron replies, "I only know the scan part." Clair begins connecting the IV port and this time the port is the correct size. Clair, "You will feel pressure in your arm for a few seconds as the radioactive tracer is being injected. Please lay still while the scan is in progress. Any questions?" Ron, "So many about the radioactive part… Let's get this over with!" The scan is completed in less than two minutes. Lamonte loads up an unsteady Ron and returns him to his room. Harry appears to be sleeping so Ron quietly changes back to his street clothes in the bathroom. Pulling on the smelly clothes reminds him to ask Patty to also pack a change of clothes with the CPAP delivery.

Inspecting his cell phone Ron notices that Patty responded and agreed to delivering the CPAP machine to the front desk and should be there within the hour. He wishes they could see each other during the delivery and dreads the thought of a long sad separation like what Harry is enduring. A blood lab cart pushed by lab tech Hermosa interrupts Ron's thoughts as she announces, "I need to gather some blood samples from you." Ron groans, "Again, I'm all out... come back next year!" Hermosa, "Doctors orders!" Two tubes of blood are drawn on the second try. The busy morning and increased abdominal pain have taken a toll on Ron. He reclines the bed for a nap.

Slumber never last long here... Ron is awakened by surgeon assistant Seeger who announces, "The scan of your lungs looks good, so we are going forward with placing a drain in your gallbladder." Ron responds, "Why not just remove it?" Surgeon replies, "There is a large amount of infection in and around the gallbladder that could contaminate other organs if we remove it now. So, we need to clear the infection up first. The procedure will be scheduled for the end of day today. The COVID patient procedures require an extensive scrub down of the operating room post use so we schedule COVID patients at the end of the day. Your nurse will let you know the time. Any questions?" Ron, "Yes, the recent lung scan confirms I don't have COVID and I am tired of being treated as such... can I get moved out of this ward?" Surgeon, "The surgery team has no control over that decision, please take it up with your assigned general physician." Ron, "What a bunch of bullshit! Then how does the drain work? Where will the infection drain to?" Surgeon, "We will insert a tube from your gallbladder to an external plastic bladder where the infection will drain into." Ron, "How long will I have this drain?" Surgeon, "The drain should remain in place for approximately three weeks and then we will reevaluate you for removing the gallbladder." Ron, "I had hoped to get this over with sooner than that! Can I eat after the surgery?" Surgeon, "You can have broth this evening and if there are no complications you will be put on solid foods starting tomorrow morning." Ron, "Thanks" Surgeon, "See you this afternoon."

## Lunch is delivered

Ron now fasting for over 81 hours receives another cup of beef broth. He removes the paper lid and gulps it down despite the disgusting taste. He notices Harry pushing his food around again, "Hey Harry, you want to sell that lunch? I haven't eaten in three and a half days!" Harry only nods and resumes messing with his food. Ron, "Yah Harry, this is one hell of a messed-up predicament!"  Harry agrees with more nods… Cassa enters the room with Ron's home CPAP bag in hand, "This just arrived for you." Ron, "Thank you!" He looks inside the bag, "Yeah, she got the message in time… a change of clothes included." He sends Patty a thank you text all the while wishing the building had better cell service to support calls. Still only one bar for cell service.

Ron unpacks the CPAP and begins setup. The hospital CPAP is huge and takes up much of the space next to his bed. Tangled in wires and tubes he carefully wheels the large cart out of the way and sets up his CPAP on the nightstand. The mask supplied by the hospital is large and better suited for use in the hospital. He attaches the larger mask to his machine and carefully climbs back into bed for a test run. Ron worries about the small filter on his CPAP. It may not be as effective for filtering out the virus as the larger HEPA filter is on the hospital machine. Ron straps the full mask over his face, "Goodbye cruel world!" He reminds himself, "I so don't want to be as sick as Harry and need to endure this safely!"

A rustling within the room awakens Ron and looking in Harry's direction finds him in a wrestling match with his blankets. Ron asks, "Harry, what's up?" No reply from Harry... Ron presses the call button. Several minutes pass and a voice asks, "Can I help you?" Ron replies, "Yes, Harry needs help with something!" A few more minutes pass and nurse tech Cassa enters the room, "Someone need help?" Ron points to Harry who has by now stopped thrashing. Cassa checks Harry's vitals and calls for assistance... he is having another panic attack. Other staff arrive and the curtain is pulled around Harry as they work on him. It takes twenty minutes for the team to get Harry stabilized. They remind him again of his need to be on a ventilator, but Harry shakes his head indicating, 'No'. The hospital staff leave the room one by one. Ron sighs, "Good grief this is ever so messed up... I must have fallen into a dark alternate universe!"

It is now 2:16 pm on Monday, which is day four for Ron, and Cassa returns to the room, "Ron you have a 4 pm appointment for a surgical procedure. Transport will be here at 3:55. Do you need anything?" Ron, "Water, thanks." Ron lays back thinking, "Now I can focus my worries on something other than dying of COVID!..." Before leaving, Cassa checks on Harry and then gives his shoulder an empathetic squeeze. Ron reclines...

## Transport Time

The blaring of the TV awakens Ron. Looking at his phone, it is 4:14pm and he is not in the operating room. He pages the nurses' station and a response asks, "Can I help you?" Ron replies, "I had a 4:00pm procedure scheduled, and transport has not arrived yet." Response, "I will check on that and get back to you." Nurse tech Cassa enters the room, "Ron, the surgery center is backed up this afternoon and your appointment was pushed to 4:45. Here is a gown that you need to put on." Ron, "Okay, thank you. I still need some water when you get a chance."

It is 4:37pm and Lamech from transport announces his arrival from the hallway. He has a rolling hospital bed for the transport vehicle. Cassa enters the room and disconnects Ron's IV and heart monitor, then pulls the curtain while asking, "Can you please get changed into the gown?" Ron responds, "Did you bring my glass slippers?" Cassa replies, "No, Just the gown." Ron greets Lamech as he steps into the hallway then climbs aboard the rolling bed.

The stress of being locked up in a COVID ward far exceeds Ron's fear of going to surgery for a procedure. The trip to the surgery center is the longest trip yet for Ron and includes a ride on a spacious elevator. His journey outside the COVID ward prompts a euphoric sensation of relief. The uplifting movement of the elevator amplifies the sensation causing Ron to grab the sides of the bed and exclaim, "Here I come lord!"

## Cold Operations

They are greeted at the surgery center by nurse tech Jewetta who directs them to the operating room. The room is extraordinarily large and cold with an equally oversized elongated table in the center. What looks like a large luggage capsule for atop a car is suspended above the table along with large lights. The room is scattered with machines on wheels and other wheeled tables. Ron exclaims, "You shouldn't have… this is too much!"

Jewetta introduces Ron to lead surgeon Dr. Cubitt and assisting surgeon Dr. Seeger. Ron, "I met doc Seeger earlier… howdy! Take it easy on me, this is my first time in an OR." Dr. Cubitt, "We will have you out of here in no time. The procedure prep work will take about fifteen minutes and placing the drain is quick, about five minutes. Then we will keep you for another 30 minutes for observation. So, the whole process will take just under an hour. Any questions?" Ron, "When can I eat?" Dr. Seeger, "Nice try, still tomorrow if all goes well." Ron, "Well have at it, but don't get your hands too close to my mouth if you want to keep them!"

Jewetta places a warming blanket over Ron and begins the prep, taking his vitals and reconnecting the IV. Jewetta asks Ron some pre-op checklist questions and Ron gets them all correct. Two shots of a local anesthetic are administered in the right side of the abdomen. Jewetta indicates they will wait a few minutes for the anesthetic to take effect.

Both surgeons are young, in their mid-twenties, and standing off to the side chatting about car stereos as Jewetta goes about completing the prep. Dr. Cubitt pinches Ron's side, "Any feeling there?" Ron, "No…" Dr Seeger lowers the imaging machine down to just above Ron's abdomen, then turns it on and begins calibration and targeting. Dr. Cubitt shows up with a long thick needle attached to a tube all inside a metal insertion tube. He inserts the needle into Ron's side and asks, "Any pain? Ron, "Nope..." Doc pushes the needle deeper and asks, "Did you feel that? I just pierced the gallbladder." Ron, "No..." Doc, "The outflow looks good, just need to secure the drain tube." The drain tube is stitched to the skin around the hose and Dr. Cubitt asks Dr. Seeger to take a look. Doc looks at the imaging screen and confirms, "It has good penetration and looks good to me."

Dr. Cubitt explains, "The drain is now in place and drains into this plastic bladder. The bladder has a twist valve on the bottom to empty the bag. You may have some minor pain around the stiches in the morning, but if you have severe pain notify the hospital staff immediately. Any questions?" Ron looks at the tube sticking out of his side and asks, "Does this really have to hang out of my body for three weeks? Dr. Seeger, "Yes, if the skin around the tube turns red call the surgeons' office." Ron, "Can I leave the hospital tonight?" Dr. Cubitt responds, "Definitely not tonight but someone from the surgery team will discuss next steps with you tomorrow." Ron, "When is dinner?" Doc Seeger chuckles, "We are out of here but Jewetta will stay here with you for another thirty minutes before we send you back to your room." Ron, "I would be fine sleeping here!" Jewetta, "Nope, cleaning crew needs to get in here and do their thing." Ron, "I just don't want to go back to that COVID ward... it is so depressing and I have no signs of COVID!" Jewetta, "Sorry, can't help you there."

The lights over the table are dimmed and Jewetta checks Ron's vitals, "Looking good." Ron asks, "Did you have the virus yet?" Jewetta, "No, thank God! They just announced today that hospital staff will be scheduled for the vaccine in just over a week from now." Ron, "You guys risk it every day and deserve to get the shots first." Jewetta, "I worry most about bringing the virus home to my family. My mother lives with us, it would be devastating if I was responsible for passing it to a family member." Ron "I hear you… I need to quarantine after I get out of here and do not know where I am going to do that. I am living in the COVID ward, but recent pre-op tests show no signs of having it. After witnessing the pain and anguish this virus causes, I would hate to give it to anyone." Jewetta, "These are some difficult times. I'm going to call transport… your thirty minutes will be up by the time they get here."

## No Running Please

Transport arrives, it is Calvin with a hospital bed. Jewetta helps Ron with his new attachment and getting onto the transport bed. Jewetta, "The drain bag has Velcro straps attached, that way it can be strapped to your leg and then baggy pants pulled over it. The hose and bag are then protected and out of the way when walking about." Ron, "Great, that sounds like a blast!" Jewetta, "No running…" Ron, "Right!" Jewetta covers Ron, "You are good to go." Ron, "Thank you for what you do!" Calvin wheels the bed out of the OR. Ron sighs, "Finally something went smoothly!"

Arriving back at the room, Ron grabs the drain bag and walks into his room, "Hi Harry, I see you haven't run off with a nurse yet!" Slumped over in his chair, Harry musters a grin. Ron takes his fresh change of clothes to the bathroom and manages to get dressed. Nurse tech Lucinda reattaches the IV and heart monitor and asks, "Do you need any pain medication this evening?" Ron responds, "No I'm okay right now thanks." Ron notices a cup of broth on his tray table then looks at Harrys tray with fish and rice half eaten and exclaims, "Harry, they are going to let me eat tomorrow!" Ron picks up the cup of broth and gulps it down exclaiming, "Tastes better every day… not!"

While examining the contents of the translucent drain bag Ron shudders, "Yuck, yeah that had to come out of there!" The bag is already one quarter filled with dark fluid. Ron starts the CPAP machine and secures the mask to his face. Ron picks up his phone… there are lots of text messages from friends and family. Ron spends the next hour texting updates to everyone and speculates, "This would be easier if I had an active Facebook account, but then it's not like I had something else to do."

Harry pushed the call button a few minutes ago but no response yet and is now banging on the call button. Ron phones the nurses' station. "Harry is having some sort of issue and needs help!" Harry is experiencing an urgent bowel movement and is in a panic over not wanting to have another embarrassing accident. Lucinda arrives and checks on Harry, then calls for assistance. Harry is moaning and breathing heavy. A few minutes later nurse tech Sanjay arrives with a bedpan. He pulls the curtain around Harry and the two techs manage to avoid a crisis this time. The odor quickly fills the room and Ron ponders, "Well, right there is one advantage I have of not eating anything! Just another day in paradise!"

Lucinda leaving the room asks, "Lights on or off?" Ron replies, "Off… but also, I asked the last shift twice for some water and didn't get any yet… can I please get some?" Lucinda returns with Ron's water and turns the light out. The TV dimly lights the room and Harry and Ron attempt some sleep. Ron sighs, "ahhh, sleeping with COVID again!"

# Chapter Five:  Let Me Out of Here

The routine morning room check awakens Harry and Ron from a deep sleep. It is Tuesday morning and Ron has one thing on his mind this morning… food! He asks for a menu. Most patients place each meal order from a small static menu. Patients too sick to do so like Harry have standing order meals sent. It is 5:34 a.m. and breakfast orders can be placed by calling the cafeteria beginning at six. Ron wants one of everything on the menu but is nutrition aware and places a bland order for oatmeal, raisins, and yogurt.

The TV is blasting the news of the latest staggering COVID infection and death numbers. Some news segments interview people with an opinion that the virus is just another virus. This virus is no joke. It takes a stay in the hospital to fully grasp the hideous lonely death by suffocation that COVID brings. There are thousands of these deaths so far and each death was slow and painful.

Harry, hunched forward in his chair, is in day 33 of a painful battle with COVID. His lost demeanor and the despairing look on his face is a tearful sight. Most of Harry's working career was spent as a union negotiator on the corporate side. He is a well-educated debater, so not being able to communicate is beyond frustrating for him.

Breakfast arrives… Ron has not eaten solid food in four and a half days and is wide eyed like a child at Christmas. The excitement soon dwindles as he tastes the cool oatmeal. Mixing in the raisins helps some. Harry received ham and eggs but has no appetite and just stares at the plate. Harry presses his call button… Nurse Trina enters the room, "Harry, what do you need?" Harry waves his hands over his untouched food motioning that he wants it taken away. Trina, "Can I get you something else?" Harry hesitates in brief thought then shakes his head indicating, 'No.' Trina asks, "Do you want to keep the coffee?" Harry places his hand on the cup and nods, 'Yes.' Trina also removes Ron's empty tray.

Ron reflects on the tube hanging from his side and slides his jogging pants down to look at the drain bag. It has a fair amount of fluid in the bag. Ron presses the call button and requests a disconnect so he can empty the bag. Nurse tech Trina enters and asks Ron, "What do you need?" Ron, "They told me to empty this drain bag frequently, it looks half full now." Trina, "I can empty that for you." Trina returns with a container. Ron, "Shouldn't this be done in the bathroom? Does it stink?" Trina, "No, here will be fine…" Trina has Ron hold the drain bag while she loosens the twist drain on the bottom of the bag. The nasty looking fluid drains into the container with surprisingly little smell. Trina takes the container to the bathroom and disposes the fluid. Ron starts to reattach the bag to his leg but notices fluid dripping from the bag onto the bed and calls out to Trina, "This thing is leaking everywhere!" Trina returns from the bathroom and tightens the drain knob while commenting, "I must not have tightened that enough. I will order you a change of sheets… sorry!"

Ella from housekeeping arrives with fresh bedding and asks, "Can you stand while I change the bedding?" Ron replies, "Sure… let me disconnect this CPAP mask." His abdomen is sore resulting in a slow-motion exit from the bed. Ella noticing Ron grimacing and asks, "Do you want a chair to sit in?" Not wanting to touch anything in the room Ron refuses the chair, though it was a good idea. Ella dislikes working in the COVID ward especially when patients are in the room. She quickly changes the bedding and exits the room.

## Culture Growth

At 9:20 Dr. Martinez from the surgery center enters… interrupting Ron's intense stare at the ceiling, with a… "Good morning!" Ron elevates the bed to a sitting position and loosens his CPAP mask to speak, "I hope it's a good morning. Can I leave the hospital today?" Doc, "What is your pain level this morning?" Ron assesses then replies, "Perhaps a nine but that is when moving and a six when laying still." Doc, "You are going to have a fair amount of pain for two to three days. We will prescribe a pain killer for that. You will not be leaving today. We still have to determine what antibiotic to send you home with." Ron, "Why does that take more than a minute?" Doc, "The lab needs to grow a culture from your gallbladder fluid to determine what bacteria we need to fight." Ron, "Grow?… How long does that take?" Doc, "About 3 days…" Ron stammers, "Oh my God! I'm not going to spend another three days in this place! My IV already has an antibiotic in it and I tolerate it, just give me that one. Pick something and release me." Doc, "Your IV antibiotic is IV specific, and I cannot send you home with an IV. I will discuss this further with the general physician, but I need to get back to the OR now."

Ron, "The abyss of hopelessness is ever expanding in this place! Just inject me with COVID and get it over with already… Damn it, I just gotta get out of here!" Surgeon Martinez leaves without further discussion. Ron, now boiling mad, moves to a meditative state attempting to defuse the rage within. He manages to unwind the spring in his head but now realizes the pain in his abdomen is severe and presses the call button to request pain medication.

Nurse Trina enters the room with Ron's pain medication and asks, "What is you pain level sweetie?" Ron replies, "Nine!" Trina administers the morphine into Ron's arm. The medication quickly reduces the pain to a tolerable level in less than five minutes. Ron picks up the menu, "What should I have for lunch?" Talking to himself seems reasonable when under the influence and when one's roommate cannot speak. He decides on a hardboiled egg with a small salad and places the order with the cafeteria.

## Dreamy Delirium Please

Moans come from Harry's side of the room. Nurse tech Aditi briskly enters the room still pulling on her protective suit. Harry's oxygen mask is detached causing low blood oxygen levels and low heart rate alarms to sound at the nurses' station. The moans stem from a dream like delirium setting in caused by the lack of oxygen. Aditi attempts to secure the mask, but Harry is confused and resisting. Head nurse Emma enters and remarks, "We need to calm him before he has another panic attack!" Both nurses begin talking to him in a soft voice while comforting him with touch. Harry relaxes and his mask is secured without further struggle. Emma leaves but Aditi stays a few minutes monitoring Harry's vitals. Harry returns to a more aware state and Aditi remarks, "Harry what are we going to do with you? Your mask needs to be on at all times!" Harry nods that he understands yet is experiencing an incomprehensible sense of hopelessness.

Eleven fifty-six and lunch is served. Harry stares at his plate for awhile but eventually eats some of his fruit cup leaving the tuna salad sandwich untouched. Ron's lunch is gone in no time. He then relaxes by texting Patty and family updates from the day. Ron receives a text from his daughter Desiree' indicating that he could come to their house for quarantine once he gets out. His daughter and son in-law both recovered from COVID several months ago. Ron agrees, it would be the quarantine option with the lowest risk to family members. They continue texting discussing the logistics.

## Treatment Options

The door opens and a distant hallway discussion is taking place. Doctor Meler a Pulmonologist and head nurse Emma enter the room. They are here to discuss with Harry his critical care options. Dr. Meler is here as a licensed pulmonologist and nurse Emma as a witness for legal safeguards.

Harry currently receives a nasal distribution of high-flow oxygen, which increases breathable oxygen. The flow is set at a maximum safe level and still not providing enough oxygen for Harry's lungs to absorb. Clinically, Harry is in respiratory distress and critically ill stemming from the coronavirus. The next progression of treatment options is the use of a ventilator. To date, Harry declined this treatment. Putting someone on a ventilator requires an informed consent and the hospital has no care consents in place for Harry. This visit is to officially document Harry's position on the ventilator use. Dr Meler must first determine if Harry has the capacity to make such decisions.

Doctor Meler is known to Harry from previous visits, "Hello Harry, I would like to discuss your condition with you, "What is your understanding of your condition?" Harry tries to speak but cannot. Nurse Emma places a pen and pad of paper in Harry's lap and squeezes his hand. Dr. Meler needs to establish that Harry is coherent and asks, "Harry, please nod 'yes' if you understand that you are critically ill stemming from the coronavirus." A frightened Harry slowly nods 'yes'... Dr. Meler, "As your pulmonologist I recommend that you be put on a ventilator. The ventilator takes over the task of breathing for you allowing the body to focus on fighting the inflammation caused by the infection. We want to take care of you in the way 'you' want to be cared for. That said, do you want to be put on a ventilator, please nod yes or no." Harry pauses in thought and shakes his head 'no'. Dr. Meler, "Is there anything we can do for you not already being done?" Harry picks up the pen and pad and writes, ' PAIN ' Dr. Meler replies, "We have you on pain medication already. I will discuss with your general physician the possibility of increasing the dosage. Anything else?" A tearful Harry writes on the pad again, "You talk my daughter?" Emma replies, "Your daughter calls often to check on you, and we provide her with updates. Is there anything you want us to tell her?" Harry writes, 'Love her – sorry'. Emma replies, "Certainly sweetie!" They conclude the counsel and leave the room. Harry sobs!

Feeling like a fly on the wall Ron contemplates, "That depressing conversation had to be a morphine hallucination! I gotta get out of here... I gotta get out of here! Alice Cooper should sing a song about that..." Ron's turbulent slumber is interrupted by the thought of food and utters, "I need to order dinner!" Ron places a dinner order for chicken, rice, broccoli, and Andre's favorite, a cookie. The cookie is denied as Ron is on a diabetic diet and cookies are not on the menu. He rejects the substitute, sugar free Jell-O… Ron hates everything that is sugar free and proclaims, "That vile tasting slime doesn't deserve to be called dessert!" Ron lays back and tries to tune out the mindless chatter coming from the TV. Thoughts of his girlfriend Patty begin providing a welcome distraction.

## Phone Visit

Dinner arrives, Harry has no appetite but manages a few sporks of mashed potatoes. Ron enjoys his dinner, savoring every bite down to the last which involves chasing a grain of rice around the plate. Ron assesses the impact of the first big meal on his starved gastric system. No change in the pain level, thereby concluding, all must be well. He pushes the tray table away and lays back looking at Harry… "Hey Harry, you saving some for later?" Harry shakes his head 'no' while pushing the table away, then presses the call button to have it removed. Ron reckons, "Harry would eat a few more bites if Emma fed it to him!" Head nurse Emma is an older nurse and Harry seems to perk up whenever she is in the room.

Emma enters the room with a pen and pad in hand. Her shift ended over an hour ago and spent the last fifteen minutes on the phone with Harry's daughter. She asks Harry, "How are you feeling Harry?" Harry knows attempting speech is fruitless and responds with a nod. Emma asks, "Your daughter would like to call, and I will mediate. Is that okay with you?" Harry nods again indicating 'Yes'. Shortly after, the room phone rings and Emma answers. Emma arranged for Harry's daughter

Cortney to call. Emma holds the phone to Harry's ear to listen to his daughter. An excited Harry writes, 'I miss you all… love you too!', which Emma communicates to Cortney. The exchange continues for a few more minutes. After they hang up Harry scrawls a large, "Thank You!!!" and shows it to Emma. As Emma leaves, Harry's thoughts bend inward reflecting on his life while raising Cortney.

11:20pm and Nurse tech Lucinda briskly enters the room followed by nurse Mary. Harry's vitals triggered alarms at the nurses' station again. Harry is slumped forward in his chair and unresponsive. Head nurse Amanda enters the room, "Get him laid back he is compressing his diaphragm!" The team reclines the chair further, causing him to lay back in the chair. Harry slowly recovers to a responsive state, but his oxygen levels remain in an alarm range. He strains to take every breath. The team leaves but Lucinda remains behind. Lucinda gets Harry to sip some water. Fifteen minutes later, Harry's oxygen level is above the alarm range and Lucinda exits the room.

The remainder of the evening is uneventful, Harry and Ron get some needed rest despite the never-ending vitals checks every three hours.

# Chapter Six:  Chilling Crash

Wednesday morning begins day six for Ron and he awakens to an urgent need for a bowel movement. Ron presses the call button for an IV disconnect. Five minutes and no response from the call for service Ron places a phone call to the nurses' station. Nurse tech Aditi informs Ron that his IV stand is on wheels and he can wheel the IV into the bathroom himself. Ron is not connected to oxygen nor the central alarm system... unlike other COVID patients he has mobility.

Ron begins the trip with the IV but realizes it is tethered to an AC wall outlet. A Tug on the cord disconnects the IV from the wall. Ron mutters, "The simple things are so cumbersome in here!" He uses the bathroom mirror to inspect the tube protruding from his side, "This is a crazy medical procedure... Frankenstein stuff!" He manages the trip to the bathroom but, plugging the IV back in is not something to be attempted as the outlet is under some equipment in use by Harry. The IV is running on battery now so Ron decides to ask someone to plug it in later.

Breakfast arrives, Harry's tray has eggs and toast... Ron a ham omelet. Harry eats just a few bites of toast dunked in egg yolk. Ron resists licking his plate and pulls the CPAP mask back on and lays back.

Nurse tech Aditi speedily enters the room. Harry's vitals alarm sounded again at the nurses' station. Harry adjusted the chair back to an upright position to eat breakfast but now asleep in a forward slump. Head nurse Emma arrives to assist with getting Harry laid back in his chair and restoring his vitals. Once laid back, Harry's vitals return to minimal levels.

## Flush with Doctors

8:45am and Surgeon Martinez enters the room and asks, "How are you feeling this morning?" Ron replies, "Physically I feel okay but suffering mentally with persistent anxiety over being in this place!" Dr. Martinez, "Well good news, I can fix that… we are going to release you today." Ron exclaims, "Yeah, can I call my ride?" Doctor, "Not yet, it will most likely be afternoon. First, a technician will explain recovery expectations and at-home care for that port we put in. Then, hospital patient administration will discuss the discharge paperwork and signatures." Ron, "Wonderful, another lunch in here."

General Physician doctor Holcomb arrives and is doing his morning rounds. He greets Harry with a "Good morning Harry." Harry responds with a weak nod. Doctor, "I see you have a request for more pain medication. I can approve a button for you to self-administer the pain medication into your IV. Do you want to try that?" Harry nods affirming 'Yes.' Harry should be in a hospice facility, but few are equipped to handle infectious disease patients. So, the hospital provides similar care in making the patient comfortable using drugs. Drugs also calm the treacherous rivers of despair. Nurse Bonnie attaches the device to Harry's IV and instructs him on the use. Dr. Holcomb listens to Harry's chest and is concerned about the level of congestion he hears and orders an X-ray to determine the lung damage progression.

Technician Dylan arrives from the Surgery Center to explain home care expectations to Ron. A five-page handout is provided describing the cleaning, antiseptic application, and protective bandaging necessary for the drain port installed in his side. Dylan reviews the handout with Ron and obtains an acknowledgment that Ron understands the care instructions. Nurse tech Sarah delivers a bag of wound dressing supplies for Ron to use at home. She also passes along a pamphlet from patient administration and indicates that someone will call to discuss the contents.

A large mobile X-ray machine is wheeled into the room. The team works on obtaining an X-ray from a barely conscious Harry. The empty hospital bed is pushed up against Ron's bed to give the X-ray team room to work around Harry's custom chair.

The vitals cart arrives pushed by Tech Anna and she announces, "I need to take your vitals." Ron responds, "I'm leaving today. Do you really need vitals?" Anna, "Yes, you are still on my rounds schedule." Ron is still shocked over the use of repeat-use oral thermometers in an infectious disease environment to gather vitals. They would not think of reusing a needle, why reuse a thermometer? Ron requests his temperature be taken from the underarm.

## Discharge Preparations

The phone at Ron's bedside rings, it is Madison from Hospital Patient Administration. Madison asks Ron to refer to the pamphlet recently delivered. She explains the discharge process and that he cannot drive himself home. She also explains the prescriptions being prescribed and contact information should he have questions. Madison asks, "Do you have any questions?" Ron replies, "What time will I be discharged? It will take my daughter an hour to get here so I would like to give her some advanced notice." Madison, "I do not have that information, please check with your nurse."

Lunch is served while Harry sleeps, dreaming of better days. Ron ordered a tuna wrap with cottage cheese. He gives the wrap two thumbs up and cleans the plate. Harry has a cookie on his tray. Ron salivates then concludes Harry must be doing better than I in the diabetes category. Harry does not eat any lunch before the tray is taken away. Ron pulls his mask on and surmises, "Well… that was a waste of a perfectly good cookie."

Ron looks at the time, 1:15 pm, and decides to give his daughter Desiree' the okay to come get him. He arranges for her to also stop and pick up some clothes from Patty, which will add twenty minutes to the one-hour trip. Ron texts other family members with the news of his imminent release and future whereabouts.

This is day six for Ron in a COVID ward and still no COVID symptoms. Sequestered in a room for six days with a virus that is killing people daily by the thousands has brought exhausting mental anguish. There are no merciful quick-death bullets flying in the COVID ward just slow lonely painful ones. This is a place where the associated delirium is a welcome distraction from the long and drawn-out pain and suffering.

Nurse tech Sarah enters and indicates, "Ron you are cleared for release and as soon as your ride arrives, I will contact transport to take you to the front door." She hands Ron some empty plastic bags and indicates, "Use these to pack anything you are taking home." Ron, "Can I keep the CPAP mask?" Sarah, "Yes, it is not reusable." Ron, "Seems inconsistent, an oral thermometer is reusable!" Sarah disconnects Ron's heart monitor and IV connections and indicates, "You need to stay in your room." Ron, "Okay, I will check with my daughter on her arrival." Ron packs his belongings then sits on the bed fidgeting with his cloth mask.

## Somber Journey

Ron texts his daughter Desiree' to determine her arrival time. She is ten minutes from the hospital. Ron asks her to let him know once at the front entrance.

Nurse tech Colleen followed by nurse Bonnie hurriedly enter the room. Harry's heart monitor triggered an alarm, so the team checks his heart rate and finds none. Nurse Bonnie calls for a crash cart. The crash cart arrives moments later pushed by nurse tech Sarah followed by Doctor Holcomb. The hospital team works on restarting Harry's heart for several minutes without success. The COVID river of doom has swept Harry away. He no longer suffers in pain and despair. The somber team disbands, and the curtain is pulled fully around Harry.

Sarah seeing a wide-eyed Ron sitting on his bed asks, "Is your ride here yet?" Ron anxiously replies, "Yes!" Sarah, "I will contact Transport." Less than a minute later Sarah re-enters with a wheelchair, "We are not going to wait for Transport. I will take you now to the front door." Ron, with a lump in his throat, gathers his belongings and is seated in the wheelchair as he tearfully gazes in Harry's direction, "Goodbye Harry!"

The journey to the front door is a somber one filled with mixed thoughts of recent despair and future hopes. Exiting the COVID ward security doors Ron imagines a change in the air quality and brighter lights which triggers an exclamation, "This must be the light at the end of the tunnel!"

Ron's daughter Desiree' awaits outside and they greet with a smile and an elbow bump. Patty also made the trip. They both wave from a distance and give each other air hugs and kisses. Desiree' hands her dad an N95 face mask and asks that he replace the cloth mask he is wearing with this one.

## Blue Skies

As they pull away from the hospital Ron grins at the bright clear day before him. He is excited like a kid traveling to Disneyland. Desiree' cannot see the smile on her dad's face and asks, "How are you feeling?" Ron replies, "I feel good… considering!" while simultaneously knocking on the dashboard. Ron, "That was a depressing ending to a way screwed-up year! But hey, being alive never felt so good! There is nothing like a terrifying hospital stay to bestow a new perspective on life!"

Ron is thankful now, but COVID may not be done with him. There is a possibility that he was infected anytime right up to the moment he left the hospital and then continue to have no symptoms for three to five days. His discharge conditions require that he quarantine for fourteen days. Desiree is giving up her home office for her dad to use as a quarantine room. After the fourteen-day quarantine

Ron must test COVID negative before he is considered not infectious.

They pass a Walgreens with a sign that reads, 'COVID-19 Testing.' Ron comments, "I need to get a COVID test as soon as possible!" Desiree' replies, "Schedule one at the Walgreens near my house. They do it using the drive-thru." Using his phone, Ron makes a 2 p.m. appointment for the following day.

The COVID test results from the following day came back as COVID negative. Ron tested again after his fourteen-day quarantine and again the test came back as COVID negative. Seems like an impossibility but Ron attributes his salvation to breathing filtered air through his CPAP machine. Ron rejoined Patty and went on to be fully vaccinated in the following weeks.

Four weeks after leaving the hospital Ron's gallbladder was successfully removed. He refused to have it done at the hospital and elected to have it done in a surgery center.

# About the Author

The author of this true story is the character Ron in the story. Born in Massachusetts and lived on the US East coast, Delmarva area, all his life. He is a military veteran and served in the Vietnam campaign. He is retired and lives in NJ with Patty.